## Praise for *Parenting Through the Storm*

"This is the first book that I've read in my long journey of parenting a child with a mental illness that didn't make me feel like I was somehow to blame. Ann Douglas actually made me feel understood and helped to stop the swirling thoughts of 'What do I do now?' In a calm and thoughtful way, she addresses so many things parents have trouble with, including self-care and caring for other children."　—Elise W., Kentucky

"This book is like having a best friend who will help you navigate the system. You'll learn what you can do to make a difference and how to know if you are getting the help your child needs. Ann Douglas is compassionate, passionate, and direct."　—Karyn D. Hall, PhD,
author of *The Emotionally Sensitive Person*

"A true gift to parents. As a mental health clinician and parent of a child who has struggled mightily over many years with major anxiety, I thought 'Hallelujah' when I finished this book. Finally, a resource that both provides validation for parents in pain and offers concrete, actionable guidance. I wish I'd had this guide when I was in the thick of it, but I am so glad it exists now, and I will recommend it to the parents I work with."　—Claire Lerner, LCSW-C, Senior Parenting Strategist,
Zero to Three

"This book fills a void in special-needs parenting resources by focusing on the big picture, and the whole family. The stories of many other parents throughout the book made me feel less alone. Reading this book, it felt like Ann was a good friend helping me through the tough times with my daughter and reassuring me that there's hope for good days ahead."
—Ashley G., North Carolina

"Raising children is tough enough, but add learning or psychological issues to the mix and no one can really prepare you for the tumultuous experience ahead. Ann Douglas does an extraordinary job of providing much-needed support, guidance, and direction. She takes you on a journey from finding out what's wrong to navigating treatment options and dealing with challenging situations. A true gem for parents!"
—Timothy E. Wilens, MD, coauthor of *Straight Talk about Psychiatric Medications for Kids, Fourth Edition*

"Ann Douglas offers hope for the many parents who are searching for answers—especially because she's been through it all herself. The book is reassuring that there's light at the end of the tunnel, but also realistic and based on research. It provides the tools you need to make tough decisions and help your child. I love this book!"   —Michele Borba, EdD, author of *UnSelfie: Why Empathetic Kids Succeed in Our All-About-Me World*

"This book is the GPS for navigating the mental health system for children and youth—period. Parents of the approximately 20% of kids who have a mental, emotional, or behavioral disorder won't want to be without it. Douglas charts a course for dealing with stigma and overcoming the shortcomings of the school and medical systems, with insight and understanding."   —Mary Gordon, Founder and President, Roots of Empathy

"An essential resource. Deeply personal and moving, this book explains the inexplicable and helps you manage your child's mental health challenges, from how to use your 'parent radar' that tells you something is amiss to getting a diagnosis and beyond. The stories of determination in these pages will shore up your courage and feed your resilience."
—Susan Newman, PhD, author of *Little Things Long Remembered: Making Your Children Feel Special Every Day*

"This is more than a book—it's a life raft for parents whose children struggle with mood disorders or developmental differences. As a parent, I've been there. You feel utterly overwhelmed by information, while at the same time isolated and without direction. Ann Douglas does something remarkable by combining concrete, empathic guidance with the voices of other parents who guide us to find the way forward."   —Asha Dornfest, author of *Parent Hacks*

# PARENTING THROUGH THE STORM

# Parenting Through the Storm

### Find Help, Hope, and Strength When Your Child Has Psychological Problems

ANN DOUGLAS

THE GUILFORD PRESS
New York     London

Published by The Guilford Press
A Division of Guilford Publications, Inc.
370 Seventh Avenue, Suite 1200, New York, NY 10001
www.guilford.com

Printed in the United States of America

This book is printed on acid-free paper.

Last digit is print number:    9   8   7   6   5   4   3   2   1

**Library of Congress Cataloging-in-Publication Data**
Names: Douglas, Ann, 1963– author.
Title: Parenting through the storm : find help, hope, and strength when your child
  has psychological problems / Ann Douglas.
Description: New York, NY : Guilford Press, [2017] | Includes bibliographical
  references and index.
Identifiers: LCCN 2016023806| ISBN 9781462526772 (pbk. : alk. paper) | ISBN
  9781462528042 (hardcover : alk. paper)
Subjects: LCSH: Mentally ill children. | Parents of mentally ill children. | Parent
  and child.
Classification: LCC RJ499.34 .D68 2017 | DDC 618.92/89—dc23
LC record available at https://lccn.loc.gov/2016023806

*To Darlene, Karen, and Lori*

*For lunches, phone calls, and emails*
*when I needed them most—at the height of the storm*

The oak fought the wind and was broken,
the willow bent when it must and survived.
—ROBERT JORDAN, *The Fires of Heaven*

And once the storm is over, you won't remember how you made it through, how you managed to survive. You won't even be sure, in fact, whether the storm is really over. But one thing is certain. When you come out of the storm, you won't be the same person who walked in. That's what this storm's all about.
—HARUKI MURAKAMI, *Kafka on the Shore*

# Contents

# Author's Note

The parent stories shared in this book are based on detailed conversations and/or correspondence with the parents who were interviewed for this new edition of *Parenting Through the Storm* or the original Canadian edition. In all cases, permission was obtained to quote these parents and to share their families' experiences. In some, identifying details were changed to protect the privacy of the individuals involved. In other cases, pseudonyms were provided at the family's request. I have edited and paraphrased some comments in the interest of clarity, while still honoring the spirit and intention of the original comments.

This book is designed to provide you with general information about child and youth mental health so that you can be a better-informed health consumer and parent. It does not contain medical advice. This book is not intended to provide a complete or exhaustive treatment of this subject; nor is it a substitute for advice from the appropriate mental health care practitioners, who know you and your child best. Seek medical attention promptly for any specific medical or psychological condition or problem that your child may be experiencing. Do not take any medication without obtaining medical advice. All efforts were made to ensure the accuracy of the information contained in this publication as of the date of writing. The author and the publisher expressly disclaim any responsibility for any adverse effects arising from the use or application of the information contained herein. While the parties believe that the contents of this publication are accurate, a licensed medical practitioner should be consulted in the event that medical advice is desired. The information contained in this book does not constitute a recommendation or endorsement with respect to any company or product.

# Acknowledgments

It would be impossible to write a book like this one without the help of a great many people.

I owe a huge debt of gratitude to the parents and other family members who agreed to be interviewed for this book: Danielle Arbuckle, Lori Bamber, Vivian Bott, Andrea Boulden, Susan Bujold, Katrina Carefoot, Sari Chateau, Danielle Christopher, Laura Devine, Shelley Divnich Haggert, Jodi Echakowitz, Darlene Evans, Rosina Fortier, Leigh Galway, Michele Girash, Christine Hennebury, Jill Jago, Laura Keller, Sandra Knof, Karen Godel Labrie, Megan Lagrotta, Jennifer Lawler, Rebecca Lee, Darlene Losier, Grace Loucks, Karen Lyall, Lisa MacColl, Stephanie MacDonald, Marie MacDonald, Kim MacKay-Hoogkamp, Cat Martin, Andrew and Eleanor Merton, Shelagh Mahri McIntyre, Micheline Miller, Mark Barranger Mitchell, Alison Palkhivala, Laurie Parr-Pearson, Cheri Patrick, Donna Pearson, Karen Petersen-Lai, Heather Petit, Laura Pettigrew, Lydia Pinkham, Tara Robertson, Marvin Ross, Susan Rvachew, Tamar Satov, Mara Shapiro, Ruby Snow, Maureen Soch, Lindalee Soderstrom, Cindy Woodcock, and the parents who chose to provide their feedback anonymously. Thank you for trusting me with your families' experiences, for sharing your hard-earned wisdom, and for your willingness to open up your hearts to help other families.

Thank you to the many mental health experts and advocates who shared valuable insights with me during the writing of this book: Darcy Gruttadaro, director of the National Alliance on Mental Illness (NAMI) Child and Adolescent Action Center in Arlington, Virginia; Ellen Leibenluft, chief of the Section on Bipolar Spectrum Disorders at the Emotion and Development Branch of the National Institute of Mental Health; Liza Long, mental health advocate and author of *The Price of Silence: A Mom's Perspective on Mental Illness*; Alison Malman, executive director and founder of the campus mental health advocacy group Active Minds, Inc.; Megan McClelland, Oregon State University developmental psychologist and coauthor of *Stop, Think, Act: Integrating Self-Regulation in the Early Childhood Classroom*; Marilyn Price-Mitchell, developmental psychologist and author of *Tomorrow's Change Makers: Reclaiming the Power of Citizenship for a New Generation*; Andrew Solomon, mental health advocate and author of *The Noonday Demon: An Atlas of Depression* and *Far from the Tree: Parents, Children and the Search for Identity*; and Joshua Weller, assistant professor of psychology at Oregon State University.

And thank you also to those equally passionate mental health experts and advocates who allowed me to interview them for the original Canadian edition of this book: Keli Anderson, president and CEO of the Institute of Families for Child & Youth Mental Health; Sarah Cannon, executive director of Parents for Children's Mental Health; Christine Cooper, executive director of the Family Association for Mental Health Everywhere; Allison Kelly, assistant professor of psychology at the University of Waterloo; Stan Kutcher, professor of psychiatry and director of the World Health Organization Collaborating Center in Mental Health Policy and Training at Dalhousie University; Lucinda Loukras, pediatrician; Walter Mittelstaedt, adjunct clinical faculty at the University of Waterloo and director of the university's Centre for Mental Health Research; Bev Ogilvie, a district counsellor with the Burnaby School District in British Columbia; Stuart Shanker, distinguished research professor of philosophy and psychology at York University and director of the Milton and Ethel Harris Research Initiative; Heather Stuart, professor of community health and epidemiology at Queen's University and the first Bell Mental Health and Anti-Stigma Research Chair; Michael Ungar, family therapist, professor of social work at Dalhousie University, and founder and co-director of the Dalhousie-based Resilience Research Centre; and Nancy L. Wolf, mental health advocate and founder of Your Bridge Forward.

Thank you to the hardworking members of the technical review panel, who went above and beyond the call of duty in their efforts to help me write the most helpful and relevant book possible: Keli Anderson; Jean Clinton, associate clinical professor in the Department of Psychiatry and Behavioral Sciences at McMaster University; Shelley Hermer, social worker at Peterborough Regional Health Centre; Catherine Kerr, early childhood consultant at Community Living Toronto; and, finally, Nancy L. Wolf, mental health advocate and founder of Your Bridge Forward, whose input into the U.S. edition of this book was truly invaluable.

Finally, I would like to thank my agent, Hilary McMahon, of Westwood Creative Artists, for believing in this project right from day one; Kitty Moore and Christine Benton, my editors at The Guilford Press, who were equally passionate champions of this project; Brad Wilson, Catherine Marjoribanks, Maria Golikova, and Stacey Cameron, my editors at HarperCollins Canada, for extraordinary editing and even more extraordinary author support; my husband, Neil, for his unwavering love and practical assistance; and my four children, Julie, Scott, Erik, and Ian, for all they have taught me—and all they will continue to teach me—about finding strength in the storm.

# Introduction

The storm has set in. Dark clouds cluster on the horizon, and the sky feels electric with change. Nothing feels the same, and yet you can't quite pinpoint what's different. Your child looks the same. Your surroundings appear the same. And yet the inner compass that guides all your parenting decisions feels like it's spinning out of control. . . .

Welcome to the club—a club you had no intention of joining, but that you find yourself a member of nonetheless: a club made up of parents who are living with the pain and worry that go along with loving a child who is struggling with a mental health challenge.

Those of us who are members of this club have certainly paid our dues, looking for help for our children and searching for answers to questions like "Why my child?"—questions that may not have answers at all.

It can make for a very lonely journey.

There may be times when you feel like you're all alone: that no one else could possibly understand what your family is going through.

The numbers, however, tell quite a different story.

Nearly one in five children and teenagers is affected by a mental, emotional, or behavioral disorder that is serious enough to cause them problems at home, at school, in the community, or in their relationships with friends.

That means a lot of kids are hurting—and a lot of families are hurting along with them.

The first step to easing that hurt is to break the silence—to reach out and connect with other families who truly understand. You'll find advice on forging those types of connections throughout this book—connections that will lend you the strength and wisdom you need to find the help your child needs.

The second step is to look for ways to make things better for your child, yourself, and your family, starting right now. That, in a nutshell, is what this book is designed to do: to launch you on your journey to a better place by giving you the knowledge you need to start making a difference for your child today.

## Why I Wrote This Book

I wrote this book in the hope of making that journey a little less lonely—and a lot less overwhelming—for you. Because the only people who can ever truly understand the pain and heartache that go along with caring for a child who is struggling with a mental health, neurodevelopmental, or behavioral challenge are other parents who have walked this path, this book relies heavily on the wisdom and experience of the brave group of moms and dads who agreed to share their stories with me. You will find their names listed in the acknowledgments.

A decade ago, I desperately needed a book like this one. Each of my four children had been diagnosed with one or more psychiatric disabilities and/or learning disabilities. I should stress that, while I'll be focusing here on the various diagnoses my four children received around the time when things were at their worst, my children are so much more than any diagnosis could ever hope to convey. DSM-5—the fifth edition of the *Diagnostic and Statistical Manual of Mental Disorders* (the mental health profession's guide to diagnosing psychiatric disorders)—may be one thick book, but it's not thick enough to capture what I love about my kids. (I'm sure you'd say the same about yours.) They're feisty, funny, opinionated people who are great to be around—and these days they're all thriving as young adults. They still face their challenges, but those up-and-down moments are nothing like the emotional roller-coaster ride we were on during their younger years. They are doing so much better than I ever could have expected—than I ever would have dared to dream—when things were at their worst.

*I know we were lucky.* Not every child or family manages to come through the storm relatively unscathed. The storm can be relentless and scarring, leaving untold damage in its wake, which is why I've chosen to round out my own experiences by sharing the experiences of other families.

But first I'm going to tell you a bit about my own experiences. And, to give you a sense of what things were like when things were at their worst for our family, I need to take you back to an earlier time, when things weren't quite so rosy—when things were actually quite awful, in fact. The year was 2003, and all four of my kids were going through a very rough time— which meant that my husband and I were going through a very rough time too. At times it felt as though our lives were falling apart. And I was about to nosedive into a deep depression that would last for a couple of years. In the interest of full mental health disclosure, I should probably tell you that I live with bipolar disorder—bipolar II to be precise, which means that I don't experience full-blown mania, but I do experience hypomania: intense, highly productive periods of creativity and high energy. I come by this bipolar thing honestly. My mother was diagnosed with bipolar I—the type with manias, including hallucinations—during my growing-up years.

Back in 2003, Julie, my oldest, was in 10th grade. She had been struggling with depression for about 2 years. The previous June, she had spent a few days in the hospital after taking an overdose of Tylenol. But now, instead of withdrawal and sadness, her depression had morphed into something angrier and much more hostile: she was climbing out the window at night so she could sneak downtown to hang out with a group of friends. She was also using drugs. What she *wasn't* doing was eating—or at least keeping food down. She had become bulimic.

Scott, who had been diagnosed with attention-deficit/hyperactivity disorder (ADHD) back in elementary school, was in ninth grade and going through the motions at home and at school. It was almost impossible to get him to follow any family rule related to computer use—actually, make that impossible. When he couldn't be on the computer, he would entertain himself by provoking his siblings, something that added to the stress and drama of family dinners.

Erik, who had been diagnosed with ADHD, oppositional defiant disorder (ODD), and a learning disability related to writing, was in seventh grade. He was having frequent outbursts—some provoked by homework or video game frustration, others provoked by Scott.

Ian, who had struggled with phonological processing disorder (difficulty making sounds) and motor-skills delays when he was younger, was experiencing a great deal of difficulty in first grade—at least in part because his teacher, who was brand new to teaching, didn't quite know what to make of him or how to manage his behavior. "I've never met a child quite like Ian," she kept telling me. He was suspended six times for a variety of offenses, including throwing a projectile object (tossing a pencil). It soon became apparent that we needed to find another school for him. We would end up trying four different schools (two public, two private) over the years before we finally found a school that was able to meet his needs. At the age of 10, he was diagnosed with Asperger syndrome, an autism spectrum disorder that is no longer a stand-alone diagnosis as of 2013,* as well as ADHD and a writing-related learning disability.

---

*The diagnosis of Asperger syndrome has been eliminated from DSM-5. Now people meeting the criteria for this disorder are simply diagnosed with autism spectrum disorder.

When things were at their worst, I remember feeling helpless and over-whelmed. I felt like a totally incompetent parent. I remember worrying about what would happen to each of my kids. I knew I had to do something to help, but what was that something?

This book is my attempt to answer that question, however belatedly.

## Who This Book Is For

There can be a great gap to cross—and a lot of learning to be done—between knowing that your child is struggling with something and coming to a full and helpful understanding of what that *something* is.

You might come to discover that your child is struggling with a psychiatric disorder or an intellectual disability, or experiencing significant psychological difficulties (for which there may or may not be a clear-cut diagnosis). Or maybe he is simply working through the challenges that are part and parcel of being a unique growing, changing, developing child. When we stop to put a name to what we see, it's a bit like stopping a movie to focus on a single frame. That single snapshot can never fully capture all of your child's strengths and weaknesses, but at least it can help to jump-start a conversation about what your child is experiencing and provide a path to treatment.

As you will see from the stories parents have contributed to this book, many children experience a cluster of different conditions: anxiety disorder plus ADHD; autism plus learning disabilities; Asperger syndrome plus obsessive–compulsive disorder (OCD). The problems are rarely simple; nor are the methods for addressing them.

What these conditions have in common is the challenge they present to these children and their families. Families are facing a storm of stress, heartache, worry, and hard work. If any of this describes your situation, then this book is for you.

## A Quick Note about Language

Language is powerful. It can also be awkward, clumsy, and just plain inadequate when it comes to describing what our families are experiencing. I tend to use the term *mental health challenges* as opposed to *mental illness* or *mental health problems* because the word *challenges* provides for greater hope and optimism: you can work to overcome a challenge. That said, language is, of course, a matter of individual choice. People need to feel empowered to use the language that best reflects their own individual circumstances and that captures both the strengths they bring to the table and the struggles they have experienced or are experiencing. So you will find the term *challenges* used extensively in this book—but you'll also find me using terms like *mental illness* or *mental health disorder* or *childhood psychiatric disorder* when describing specific psychiatric conditions. Ditto for the term *neurodevelopmental disorder*, because sometimes that term can be helpful in pinpointing exactly what we're talking about. And, of course, you'll find me using the term *mental health* to describe the state of being mentally healthy. As the World Health Organization points out, mental health is not merely the absence of mental illness. Mental health is about thriving. It is important to acknowledge that mental health and mental illness are not mutually exclusive. It is possible to experience mental health while living with mental illness. That is what the mental health recovery movement is all about: maximizing mental health while living with a mental illness.

But enough about terminology. You're probably wondering what this book is all about and how to zero in on the information that is most relevant to you right now. Here's what you need to know.

## How to Navigate Through This Book

This book is divided into five parts, which will guide you through a widening perspective on the challenge you are facing with your child, with your family, and in your community.

Part I looks at the tools you will need to get started in finding help for your child and making things better. You will find guidance for interpreting the symptoms when your "parent radar" is telling you something might be wrong; advice on the process of diagnosis; information about treatment options; and direction for your efforts as your child's most important advocate. But this book is also about you—your worries, your stresses, your feelings—so all along the way you will find advice from other parents and useful information to help you get the support you need.

In Part II you will read more about what you are going through in your relationship with your child. You will find tips on reducing stress so that you can safeguard your own mental health and advice on maintaining your loving connection with your child while you help him learn how to manage his emotions and his behavior more effectively.

In Part III the focus broadens to look at your experience with your child in the context of your family as a whole—because you are all going through this together! You will also read about some recommendations for changes you might want to make to your lifestyle that will help the whole family feel better physically, mentally, and emotionally.

Part IV takes you out into your community, discussing the challenges that might come up for your child at school and with friends, including the issue of bullying. And you will read about ways to find support for yourself from the people around you and the people you work with.

Part V looks at the idea of recovery, which basically means living the best possible life in the wake of particular challenges—the successes and the setbacks and new dreams for the future—and what that might mean for your child, for you, and for your family and community. And finally, we'll look at ideas for a better system of care for children with mental health, neurodevelopmental, and behavioral challenges, and what you might be able to do to help make that a reality.

As always, I would welcome your comments and input for future editions of this book. You can send your comments to me online via my website, *www.anndouglas.net*.

Best wishes to you, your child, and the rest of your family as you weather the storm together.

# Part I

# The Challenge
# and Your Child

If your child is struggling with psychological problems and challenges—at this point, early in your journey, it may still feel strange to see that written out in black and white—you are likely struggling yourself, feeling frightened and alone, uncertain about how to help your child or where you can turn for the information and support you so desperately crave. If you grew up with a family member who struggled with mental health challenges, you may be heartbroken and terrified about what the future may hold for your child.

It's easy to lose your sense of direction during the peak of the storm, to stumble, to get lost. That's what this first part of the book is for: to help you make your way through the chaos and the confusion and arrive at your destination. In this section of the book, we will deal with some of the important steps to take toward getting help for your child from the health care system: assessing symptoms, obtaining a diagnosis, navigating treatment options, and advocating for your child all along the way. This can all be very daunting, but there is a lot of support out there for you, and hopefully the information here will provide a helping hand.

Connecting with other parents who truly understand is an important first step, which is why you'll be encountering so many parent stories in the first part of the book. You need to know that other parents have made it through, and that you have the courage and strength you'll need. There were times when I wondered how I would find that courage and that strength myself. And yet I did because I had to. My children were counting on my husband and me to do everything we could to guide them through the storm.

The storm struck for us when my daughter was 13 and going through a very dark time. She had been struggling with depression for over a year and, at some point during the final months of eighth grade, she stopped being able to imagine life ever getting any better. In an effort to make the pain go away, she took a large quantity of Extra Strength Tylenol.

We were lucky. I found her in time and recognized that something was wrong. We spent that night in intensive care, me holding the baby-blue vomit basin up to her mouth as the activated charcoal worked its magic, soaking up the toxins in her stomach.

While she slept fitfully for 45-minute stretches at a time, in between spasms of vomiting, I stretched out on the three metal-framed chairs that a kindhearted nurse had assembled into a make-shift bed for me.

I thought back to an earlier time, when I was a brand-new mother up in the middle of the night in this very same hospital with this very same child, then a tiny newborn. I remembered how scared and uncertain I had felt during those early hours and days of motherhood.

Those same feelings were back once again. But this time, there weren't any mom-and-baby classes I could take to tell me how to keep my teenage daughter safe from herself.

It didn't matter that I was in the heart of a busy hospital, surrounded by the hustle and bustle of the ICU, and just inches away from my sleeping daughter. I felt utterly, totally alone. I felt like my daughter was slipping away.

We made it through that crisis and the countless others that followed over the next few years—crises that necessitated trips to the emergency room; calls to police officers; and appointments with social workers, psychiatrists, and other experts. And so did Julie. As I write this book, she is a healthy 27-year-old and a talented young artist with a passion for abandoned places and anything else whose beauty has been overlooked by the rest of the world.

Kids can come through the worst of times. So can families. We're a resilient lot. (Thankfully.)

You'll pick up on that spirit of resilience as you make your way through the first part of this book, which is largely a tapestry of other parents' stories. You will notice that, even while parents are speaking of the wrenching pain they endured while their children were struggling, their love and commitment to their children shine through. It all begins with love.

> Looking back over a lifetime, you see that love was the answer to everything.
>
> **Ray Bradbury**

# 1

# Parent Radar

Our instincts tell us when something's not right with our kids. We place a hand on a toddler's forehead if she seems more lethargic than usual and ask ourselves, "Could she be coming down with a fever?"

In the same way, parent intuition can alert us to the symptoms of a psychological problem. In this case, it's a child's behavior rather than a spike in temperature that causes us to become concerned. If only we had a mental health thermometer in our medicine cabinets.

"The doctor was amazed that I picked up on the signs so early," recalls Lisa, whose daughter, Laura, has been struggling with behavioral issues at home and at school and is currently awaiting diagnosis. "But she's my child and I know her better than anyone."

You may be reading this book because you're worried about your child. You may be wondering if the behavior you've noticed lately is something all children go through—or is it a symptom of something more worrisome? You may find yourself wavering back and forth on this question, sometimes thinking yes and sometimes thinking no, and sometimes feeling unsure. You may feel like your parent radar is permanently stuck in the worry zone, but you're not quite sure why.

> You know your child better than anyone. The most important tool you have is your instinct.
>
> **Mark, father of Dawson, who has been diagnosed with reactive attachment disorder, anxiety disorder, and moderate developmental disability**

# Why You May Be Worried

## Those First Moments of Worry

Some parents can date their first nagging concerns back to when their children were still babies.

"With Aiden, I knew something was wrong from when he was an infant," recalls his mother, Tara. Aiden has since been diagnosed with autism and ODD. "He just never stopped crying. He would cry for 10 or 11 hours a day, every day. That continued until he was almost 1 year old. Doctors told me he was just really colicky. He was also really, really active; and the older he got, the more violent he got. He would throw himself into things: the couch, the wall, the floor."

Karen, whose son Spencer was diagnosed with pervasive development disorder not otherwise specified (PDD-NOS),* had a similar experience: "I remember Spencer being 8 months old and having tantrums that were so violent he would bang his head on the floor until he vomited. The more I tried to subdue him, the more his rage escalated. I knew that this was outside the range of normal. Our doctor brushed off my concerns by saying, 'He'll grow out of it.' Actually, he grew into it, and as he got bigger, the rage got bigger too." It was only after Karen insisted on a referral to a developmental pediatrician that things started to get better for her son: "He was the first person to agree that there might be an issue other than the terrible twos."

## School-Related Worries and Concerns

Other parents don't notice any worrisome symptoms until after their child has started school.

"I first began to suspect that there was an issue when Will was constantly sent home from first grade for uncontrollable behavior," recalls Christine, his mother. "When Will was suspended in second grade for hurting another child, we knew for sure that there was an issue." A short time later, Will was diagnosed with severe ADHD and an anxiety disorder.

"Skyler had always been a happy child, but that changed fairly significantly when he ran into the 'wall' of the structure and expectations of school," recalls Leigh, whose son has been diagnosed with ADHD, anxiety, and depression. "The things he normally liked to do became frustrating for him and he retreated into himself. When forced to engage with

---

* The diagnosis of PDD-NOS, like that of Asperger syndrome, has been eliminated from the fifth edition of the *Diagnostic and Statistical Manual of Mental Disorders* (DSM-5) and replaced by "autism spectrum disorder."

others in a context in which he was uncomfortable, he would become quite agitated and respond in inappropriate ways. We sought professional help when Skyler was 6 years old. He had been suspended from school for an incident involving frustration tolerance and self-control and, as a result, he attempted suicide."

## Triggering Events

Some parents can pinpoint a particular event that seemed to trigger a child's difficulties. Kate remembers her son Tony showing signs of depression in the aftermath of his father's death. He was just 7 years old at the time. "He would cry at night, after the first year, that he was forgetting his dad."

More often than not, however, there isn't any clearly identifiable trigger. A cluster of worrisome symptoms develops over a period of time. Or a crisis occurs, demanding immediate attention.

## The Frequency of Symptoms

It might not be the symptom alone but the frequency of the symptom that suggests a problem. For example, although many preschoolers are given to temper tantrums, the frequency and intensity of tantrums in children of that age may be a warning sign of a possible problem. A study published in a 2012 issue of *The Journal of Child Psychology and Psychiatry* reported that while 80% of preschoolers had thrown one or more temper tantrums in the previous month, fewer than 10% of preschoolers threw tantrums on a daily basis. What's more, the researchers found that there was more likely to be cause for concern if children had a temper tantrum when they were being cared for by an adult who was not their parent, if they destroyed objects during a tantrum, if there was no apparent reason for the tantrum, if the tantrum was prolonged, or if the preschooler became violent during the tantrum (hitting, biting, or kicking someone else).

A child who is experiencing severe tantrums may end up being diagnosed with an impulse control disorder. According to research conducted by the National Institute of Mental Health (NIMH), impulse control disorders have the earliest age of onset of all the psychiatric disorders, with onset typically occurring between the ages of 7 and 15. ADHD (which is also considered to be a neurodevelopmental disorder) tends to become a problem during the primary school years. ODD, conduct disorder, and intermittent explosive disorder (behavioral disorders) tend to show up a little later on, during the preteen and teen years. Note: Some children with extreme irritability and severe tantrums meet the criteria for a brand-new diagnosis—disruptive mood dysregulation disorder (DMDD). It was added to DSM-5 to describe children who would otherwise meet the criteria for a bipolar diagnosis except for the fact that they aren't subject to manias or hypomanias.

Anxiety disorders also tend to have their onset during childhood and adolescence, typically between the ages of 6 and 21. Phobias and separation anxiety disorder tend to be a problem for younger children, while other types of anxiety disorders, such as panic disorder, generalized anxiety disorder, and posttraumatic stress disorder (PTSD), tend to be more of a problem for slightly older children and teens.

Alison chose to seek help for her daughter, Charlotte (who was ultimately diagnosed with an anxiety disorder), after noticing a pattern of worrisome behaviors. "She had several symptoms that together made me concerned: a tendency to scratch at her face, nail biting, chewing at her clothes and anything else she could get her hands on, difficulty with separating at night, difficulty sleeping, difficulty sleeping on her own, and an unwillingness to participate in [Girl Scout] activities outside of the regular weekly meeting, even though she loves [Girl Scouts]."

Other types of disorders begin to show up during the teen years. Mood disorders become more prevalent starting in the early teens, and substance abuse disorders and eating disorders become more of a concern starting in the midteens. Psychotic disorders rarely occur before age fourteen but become significantly more prevalent between the ages of 15 and 17. And personality disorders, which involve an enduring pattern of distress and difficulty functioning, are typically diagnosed during adolescence or early adulthood.

### Changes in Behavior

Joanne, whose son William has been diagnosed with major depressive disorder (MDD), a type of mood disorder, sprang into action after noticing some troubling changes in her son's behavior. "William started hanging around with a different group of friends," she recalls. "He came home drunk for the first time at age 15. His art and drawings were all of a sudden private. When I found his art book, I discovered that the drawings had become very dark; the style had changed completely. He was drawing faceless boys, cut and bleeding, decorated—I suspected—with real blood. He started writing out lyrics to sad and violent songs. He stopped being able to sleep at night or get up in the morning. He started challenging my husband at every turn. He stopped doing his homework. This all happened very quickly. He was not the same person. I took him to our doctor for an assessment."

Andrew, whose son David has been diagnosed with schizophrenia, recalls a similar downward spiral. "Around ninth grade, David began to skip classes. He was hanging around with a friend who seemed to have a disregard for adult authority. Later, we found out that substance use—marijuana, cough syrup concoctions—was also beginning to happen. Things went missing and were likely sold to get substances. In 10th grade, David became more angry and withdrawn. He was beginning to show signs of verbal aggression as well and this was quite disturbing as it seemed so alien in our household, given the values we tried to pass on as parents . . . Around this time, there were also a couple of violent situations where David struck me in moments of conflict."

Sometimes the signs that a young person is struggling aren't immediately apparent. A young person may engage in self-harm without anyone knowing. Self-harm may involve self-injury (cutting, burning, stabbing, running out in front of cars), self-poisoning (overdosing on medication or consuming toxic substances), and risk-taking or otherwise health-harming behaviors (substance abuse, food restriction, unsafe sex).

Self-harm is more common than most people realize. A study of non-suicidal self-injury rates in children and youth ages 7 through 16 found that 9% of girls and 6.7% of boys had self-injurious thoughts and/or engaged in self-injurious behaviors. The study, which was published in the July 2012 issue of the medical journal *Pediatrics,* noted that ninth-grade girls were most at risk and that they were most likely to resort to cutting themselves as a means of self-injury.

The incidence of suicidal thinking and behavior is even more disturbing. Researchers have found that one in four adolescents reports suicidal thoughts or attempts and that there is a peak in suicidal thinking between the ages of 14 and 18 years. And, tragically, those thoughts can all too easily translate to action: according to NAMI, suicide is the second-leading cause of death in young people ages 15 through 24 and the third-leading cause of death in children and youth ages 10 through 24.

These statistics may leave you feeling frightened and helpless—but you don't have to feel that way. There are things you can do to reduce the likelihood that your child will attempt suicide. The most powerful things you can do are to consistently stress how much you value your child's life (sometimes suicidal people think they will be doing friends and family members a favor by taking their own life because they feel that they have become a burden to others), help your child develop resiliency and coping skills (be in good physical and psychological health, know when and how to ask for help), and help your child develop a solid network of support (support from family and friends, access to community supports). Don't be afraid to talk to your teenager about suicide for fear of planting the idea in his head. He will be safer if he knows that he can come to you to talk about whatever is on his mind, even his darkest and most despairing thoughts. Besides, not talking about suicide doesn't make suicidal thoughts go away. It simply drives those thoughts underground.

Dawne knew it was time to act on the nagging doubts she had been harboring for a while about her son Peter's behavior when he threatened to harm himself. Peter was subsequently diagnosed with a nonspecific pervasive personality disorder with some characteristics similar to Asperger syndrome (a condition now diagnosed as autism spectrum disorder), as well as anxiety. "When he was nine, he had a really bad meltdown in which he threatened to cut his throat with a knife," she recalls. "That's when I knew he needed help. I called a number for a counseling service I had been considering and, when I told them what he'd said, they told me to take him to the hospital right away."

### When Others Raise the Alarm

Sometimes, it's a third party who alerts a parent to the fact that there's a serious problem.

That's how Micheline discovered that her son Sean, who has been diagnosed with ADHD after an earlier diagnosis of anxiety and OCD, had been cutting himself. "When he was 13, we were called by the principal, who indicated she had heard from a friend of Sean's that he was cutting the tops of his thighs. We looked him over and were heartbroken. There were several fresh marks as well as scars."

## The Feeling That Something Is Wrong

Sometimes it's our own nagging feeling that something isn't right that motivates us to dig a little deeper—to find out what's really going on.

That's how things played out for Lily and her daughter, Asia, who was ultimately diagnosed with borderline personality disorder (BPD): "One evening, my daughter was supposed to be at a friend's house and I was planning to go out for dinner," Lily recalls. "For some reason—perhaps I'd forgotten something—I returned home. As soon as I got in the house, I had a feeling my daughter was there and that something was terribly wrong. Perhaps I'd heard something without being conscious of it, or perhaps 'mother's intuition' really exists. Either way, I started searching for her—searching rooms and then, when I didn't find her, searching under beds and in closets. I found her in a closet, covered in her own blood. She'd been slashing her arms with a knife after someone she thought was a friend had rejected her. She wasn't crying, just trembling like she was chilled, in shock. That was when I knew that we needed help. Before then, she had told me about her feelings of hopelessness and anxiety, and I had chalked it up to being a teenager—partly because I had experienced the same feelings at the same age. It would be another couple of years before I realized that I was mentally ill as a teenager as well. In those days, it was just called *rebellion*—being a bad kid."

It's hard not to blame yourself if you feel like you missed some clues that might have encouraged you to seek help for your child sooner rather than later. It may be helpful to remind yourself that you did the best you could with the information you had at the time. What more can we ask of ourselves, really?

As these stories suggest, the symptoms of mental illness are different in children than they are in adults and can differ depending on age and stage of development. Children are constantly changing—and their circumstances are constantly changing too. A lot of teenagers who wouldn't meet the diagnostic criteria for any disorder still manage to exhibit a lot of very worrisome symptoms—symptoms that may ebb and flow as a child matures or situations change. This can make it difficult to pinpoint the nature of a particular mental, emotional, or behavioral disorder in a particular child. On pages 18–19 are some symptoms you should be alert to.

If your parent radar is telling you to be concerned, then some follow-up is called for. While you are the expert on your own child, other people have expertise, experience, and perspectives that might be helpful too. What you're looking for is evidence that your child's behavior is interfering with her ability to function—and what you're witnessing goes beyond a single bad day.

## What Can You Do If You Are Worried That There May Be a Problem?

### Talk to Other People

You might want to start with other people who know your child well: this could include other family members, your child's teachers or coaches, and close friends of the family—people whose opinion you trust. Ask if they have noticed the same or other worrisome symptoms or behaviors in your child. You can start these types of conversations with a simple question, such as "Do you think I need to worry about Jason's temper tantrums?" or "Do you think I should be concerned about Rachel's crying spells?"

## The Warning Signs of Potential Mental Health Problems in Children and Adolescents

A checklist based on the following is available to be downloaded at *www.guilford.com/douglas-forms* and can be kept with your child's records.

### In Infants

- Your baby doesn't turn to you for comfort.
- Your baby doesn't demonstrate affection.
- Your baby ignores you, avoids you, or demonstrates a lot of anger after you've been away from her.
- Your baby doesn't seem interested in "talking" with people or making eye contact.
- Your baby is just as affectionate with strangers as she is with people she knows well—and she has reached the age (8 to 18 months) at which stranger anxiety typically becomes a problem.
- Your baby doesn't look to you for reassurance when she is exploring her environment (a behavior known as *social referencing*, which typically emerges at around 9 months old) *or* your baby doesn't explore her environment at all.
- Your baby doesn't seem to understand that he can turn to you for help.
- Your baby doesn't seem to understand that she can do some things on her own.

### In Children and Teenagers

- Your child is having more difficulty at school.
- Your child is hitting or bullying other children.
- Your child is attempting to injure himself.
- Your child is threatening to run away.
- Your child is avoiding friends and family.
- Your child is experiencing frequent mood swings (mood swings that seem to be something more than the moment-to-moment shifts in mood that are typical of the teenage years).
- Your child is experiencing intense emotions (extreme fear, angry outbursts).
- Your child is lacking in energy or motivation.
- Your child is no longer pursuing hobbies or interests he used to enjoy.
- Your child is having difficulty concentrating.
- Your child is having difficulty sleeping or having a lot of nightmares.
- Your child is experiencing a lot of physical complaints.
- Your child is neglecting her appearance.

- Your child is obsessed with his weight, shape, or appearance.
- Your child is eating significantly more or less than usual.
- Your child is consuming a lot of alcohol or using drugs—or your child is experimenting with alcohol before reaching high school age.

---

*Note.* Your child may exhibit one of these symptoms or a number of symptoms. You know your child best. What you are looking for are changes in your child's usual behavior or a discrepancy between the types of behaviors you would expect to see in a child at a particular developmental stage and what you are observing in your child. Don't forget to take into account other factors that can have an impact on your child's social and emotional development, at least over the short term: being born prematurely, losing a primary caregiver or experiencing another similarly traumatic event, or having a history of significant medical interventions.

*Sources:* Data from *KeltyMentalHealth.ca*, "What Is Infant Mental Health?"; *Kidsmentalhealth.ca*, "Mental Health Disorders in Children and Youth: Identifying the Signs"; National Institute of Mental Health, "Treatment of Children with Mental Illness."

## *Talk to Your Child*

You might want to talk to your child, depending on her age, about your concerns. Ask your child how she is feeling these days. Let your child know that you care, and ask what you can do to help. If you're concerned that your child could be experiencing suicidal feelings, confront the issue directly. Ask your child, "Do you ever have thoughts and feelings about death?" "Do you ever wish that you wouldn't wake up or that everything (and everyone) would go away?" If your child admits to having such feelings, resist the temptation to hit the panic button yourself and to seek immediate reassurance from your child that she wouldn't actually follow through on those feelings. Saying something like "But you'd never actually hurt yourself, right? You know what that would do to your family" will only make your child feel bad for worrying you and encourage her to hide her feelings from you in the future. It doesn't deal with the underlying problem. A better approach is to acknowledge what your child is saying, to let your child know that you care, and to make a commitment to seek help: "I am sorry you are feeling so bad. I love you. We're going to get you some help."

Of course, if your child is expressing suicidal thoughts, it is important to seek help immediately, by heading for the closest hospital (ideally one that has a pediatric psychiatric unit, if there is one in your area) or by calling 911 (if you are dealing with a crisis situation). Peer support is critical for teenagers, so you may want to ask your teenager if he would like to take a friend with him to the assessment, if you're heading for the hospital. If your child is in crisis and you don't feel that it would be safe for you to attempt to take your child to the hospital yourself, call 911 and ask for a police

officer trained in mental health (ideally one who has taken crisis intervention training to learn how to deescalate situations in which an individual is
extremely agitated and potentially violent).

### See a Doctor

Set up an appointment to discuss your concerns and to have your child
assessed by his pediatrician or other primary care provider. The doctor
either will be able to assess your child or will refer your child to another
health care professional or agency for a more comprehensive assessment.
(See Chapter 2 for more detailed information about obtaining a diagnosis
for your child.) Having your child assessed by a health care professional can
also help identify and address any medical conditions that might be contributing to your child's distress. Ann's daughter Eleanor exhibited extreme
behavior as a means of coping with debilitating physical pain from her
digestive disorder. "She would be asking for something that was physically
impossible," Ann recalls. "She spent 3 hours one day screaming at me to
put her boots on so that we could go to the park *when her boots were already
on.* And when I tried to take her boots off so that I could put them back on,
she kicked me in the face."

### Speak Up

This is where your input becomes extremely valuable. You can zero in on
worrisome changes you may have noticed in your child's behavior—they
could be the symptoms in the checklist on pages 18–19, or anything else
that your gut instinct is telling you to pay attention to. Make a point of raising these issues with your child's doctor.

Spend some time preparing for your child's initial consultation. You
can help the person who is conducting the assessment—your child's pediatrician or a specialist in children's mental health—to decide whether or
not there is cause for concern (and whether additional referrals or a full
assessment should be recommended) by jotting down a few notes about
your child's symptoms and behavior and taking these notes with you to
your child's appointment. The purpose of a mental health assessment is to
answer two key questions: Does this child have a disorder and, if so, what
is the correct diagnosis? The person conducting this assessment will rely on
the information you and your child are able to provide: your responses to
questionnaires and rating scales, existing information that provides insights
into your child's functioning and psychological health (for example, report
cards and the results of any psychological or educational testing conducted
to date), an observation of your child's behavior, and interviews conducted

with both your child and you. The more information you can provide about your child's academic achievement, relationships (both within the family and with friends), leisure activities, and level of functioning and self-care, the more accurate the resulting diagnosis will be.

In preparation for your appointment, you may want to make note of:

- The types of symptoms that your child is exhibiting (and how long and how often he has been exhibiting these symptoms), and whether you have noticed any sudden changes in his level of functioning.
- Whether you've noticed any particular patterns associated with these symptoms (times of day and any suspected triggers).
- The types of settings that are the most difficult for your child.
- Any events or circumstances that may have contributed to your child's difficulties (if applicable)—perhaps situations of change, grief, or loss, or an incident that was traumatic for your child.
- How you have tried to help your child (both what's worked and what hasn't worked). What parenting strategies have you tried at home? What types of programs and services have you accessed in an effort to support your child? What medications have been tried?

Try to obtain your child's input into these questions, both so that you can gain valuable insights into what he is thinking and feeling and so that you can encourage him to play an active role in managing his own mental health, right from day one. And be sure to let your child know that he is not alone in dealing with these challenges. You will be there for him because you care.

Make this information the first entry in a journal you use to keep track of your child's symptoms and behaviors. You'll also want to start a binder to keep track of correspondence with health care providers, copies of assessments and other documents related to your child's treatment history, copies of report cards, and other information that you will want to be able to access quickly and easily. See Chapter 4 for more advice on what to store in the binder, how to connect with parent support groups, and how to advocate for your child.

> Focus less on the diagnosis and more on helping your kid with whatever symptoms he or she is facing right now. . . . At every appointment with every clinician, bring up the issue of treatment. What can we do right now to help my child while the assessments are ongoing? Focus on what is really making your child suffer and be a broken record about it. You need help now with these symptoms. You can't wait.
>
> **Alison, mother of Charlotte, who has been diagnosed with an anxiety disorder**

## How You May Be Feeling

The early days when you first begin to suspect that your child may have a mental health or developmental challenge tend to be particularly stressful. You still don't know for certain what your child is dealing with, so it's too soon to channel your emotions into action. This can leave you feeling anxious, frustrated, and helpless. You may feel as though your entire life is on hold while you wait for answers.

That was certainly the case for Christine, mother of Will. "Prediagnosis, before I understood what was going on, my mental health definitely suffered," she recalls. "I was constantly anxious, didn't sleep, didn't have time for exercise, and stopped seeing friends and extended family. I just didn't have the energy or strength to deal with what Will was going through and to maintain friendships at the same time. I became very isolated, with my husband and my children being the only people I saw most days. I quit volunteering at the school because it was too stressful to see Will struggling so much in the classroom and with his peers. I work as a freelance writer and editor from home and, for the first time ever, I had to quit a stressful job in the middle of it because I couldn't handle the additional anxiety. I permanently damaged my relationship with that client. I also cut back on my hours, from 35 hours per week to about 25. I just felt that I was dealing with too much to continue working full-time."

Mark, whose son Dawson was diagnosed with reactive attachment disorder, an anxiety disorder, and moderate developmental disability 5 years after his adoption, recalls a time when his son's mental illness became the sole focus of his life: "There was a long period of time—probably about a year in length—when I couldn't focus on anything else. I had to be ready to drop everything if Dawson needed me. It was the hardest year ever. I took a leave of absence from my job at one point because I couldn't concentrate on anything other than what was going to get my son through this."

Leigh, mother of Skyler, can relate to those feelings—feelings that continued as her son moved into the diagnosis and treatment phase. "Providing the required emotional support for a child with mental health issues is exhausting for a parent. *Exhausting*," she explains. "I felt like I was on 'hyper-alert' all the time, just waiting for the next incident. I was overwhelmed with the need to schedule appointments with pediatricians, psychologists, psychiatrists, and so on. It consumed my life. Everything else took a back seat: my marriage, my older son, my work, my extended family. It was easier to shut down and just deal with what was happening at any particular moment."

Feelings of exhaustion quickly become the new normal.

"I haven't slept through the night since my son was born 11 years ago," says Tara, mother of Aiden, and of Owen, who has been diagnosed with anxiety and ADHD. "I am on medication for depression. I am overweight because I stress-eat and self-medicate with food. Ice cream is my drug of choice."

"Sophie has sleep issues, and often, as many as two nights a week, she will have me awake from 2 to 5 A.M.," says Sandra, her mother. Sophie was diagnosed as having moderate autism with global developmental delays. "Yet we still get up at 7 to start our day. It affects the rest of my day, being tired, not having energy to work out, eating poorly to try to get extra energy."

"Adam often wakes us up during the night and early mornings," says his mother, Tami. Adam has been diagnosed with ADHD. "Sometimes he will go downstairs at 4 A.M. and turn on the TV, and we have to go tell him to go back to bed. Sometimes he rages and throws things or slams doors. Because I do not function well without sleep, I often end up going to bed around 9 P.M., shortly after Adam does, which cuts into my alone time with my husband."

Other common emotions include grief, anxiety, guilt, sadness, and anger.

"I am feeling a lot like I did when Veronica first fell ill as a toddler: a lot of uncertainty and fear for the future—no guideposts, no moorings either. Drifting in a sea of grief and anxiety," says Sarah, whose daughter has been diagnosed with Asperger syndrome and an anxiety disorder.

"Because my son had made a suicide attempt, I was terrified," recalls Leigh, mother of Skyler. "I remember wondering, 'Can I leave him alone? Do I have to put my house on lockdown? Do I need to hide every sharp object? What about the car keys? Can I sleep? Is he safe?' Anxiety became my new life partner."

"We have suffered depression ourselves because we have felt like failures," says Owen's mother, Claire, whose son—now a young adult—has been diagnosed with bipolar disorder, a personality disorder, and extreme anxiety. "We have felt hopeless at times because mental illness does not go away. It is something you will be dealing with for the rest of your child's life. It has made me feel jealous of families who seem to have no issues."

> Remember, when you are feeling sorry for yourself because it's hard to have a child with mental illness, that it's even harder to be a child with mental illness.
>
> **Michelle, whose son John was diagnosed with depression with suicidal thoughts and whose son Martin was diagnosed with generalized anxiety disorder**

"I emotionally died for some time," says Jackie, whose two sons, David and John, have been diagnosed with psychosis. "I went into mourning: I mourned for everything they had lost—the life they probably would not have anymore."

Mark, Dawson's father, has struggled with a lot of anger. "I am so angry about what was done to my son before we adopted him," he explains. "I am angry at the system that took so long to diagnose him—that took that much time away from him and his life. I guess if I really think about it, I am angry at myself too. I sometimes feel that what I can do isn't enough."

It's not unusual to experience a smorgasbord of emotions, sometimes at the same time. You may feel pushed to your limits and beyond—a feeling that Lisa, mother of Laura, readily admits to experiencing: "I have found patience I never knew I had. I have also, sadly, found depths of anger I never thought I was capable of when Laura's pushing the last button and it's 10 P.M."

> It's not unusual for us to become frustrated, irritated, and impatient at times with the behaviors that now seem to be typical. For example, David can become rude and demanding very quickly. He escalates into anger very easily, and his ability to reason is quite limited. He does not seem to be aware of social etiquette. This can create awkward situations. On the one hand, we are sympathetic to the way schizophrenia impairs him socially and emotionally, but at times we treat him as if he should know better. It's a tricky balance because, to some degree, he can improve some of his behavior, but, overall, he seems to have a certain baseline of functioning that is dictated by the illness. We know that being informed and staying informed about the illness keeps us better aware of what to expect and thus how to best respond. Sometimes our less than desirable responses are likely connected to our own grief and anger about seeing our child afflicted with a horrible illness and knowing his future is very altered because of that. Being self-aware, often helped by talking to a professional, has enabled us to not confuse our own baggage with our feelings about our child.
> **Andrew, father of David, who has been diagnosed with schizophrenia**

## Taking Care of Yourself

It may seem self-indulgent to think about taking care of yourself when your child is struggling with a mental or developmental challenge. After all, shouldn't your child be your top priority—your only priority—right now?

Actually, *you* need to be your top priority, because, without you, your child will be lost.

"Doing something for yourself to make sure you can cope is as important for your child's well-being as doing something directly for the child," insists Sandra, mother of Sophie.

Marie, whose son David has been diagnosed with the severe combined form of ADHD, sensory integration disorder, and two learning disabilities (one in math and one in writing), agrees. "Take care of yourself," she insists. "If you don't, you can't help anyone else."

So what does it mean to take care of yourself? Here are a few gifts you can give yourself that will end up benefiting everyone in your family.

### Find Acceptance

Accept your situation for what it is, so that you can begin to work within that reality. A study related to autism conducted by researchers at York University and the Centre for Addiction and Mental Health in Toronto, Canada, concluded that "for problems that are chronic and difficult to address, psychological acceptance may be an important factor in coping for parents of young people" with autism spectrum disorder. Likewise, Pat Harvey and Jeanine A. Penzo, coauthors of *Parenting a Child Who Has Intense Emotions: Dialectical Behavior Therapy Skills to Help Your Child Regulate Emotional Outbursts and Aggressive Behaviors*, suggest that parents focus on accepting their child for who she is while, at the same time, working on behaviors that are a challenge to both of you—and that they extend the same spirit of kindness and compassion to themselves. "You and your child are doing (and have done) the best that you can, *and* you can both learn new skills to do even better," they write.

### Give Forgiveness

You're not perfect, and you don't have all the answers. You can forgive yourself for being a gloriously imperfect work in progress, just like your child. This sure beats being unkind to yourself for not being able to meet your own impossible and unrealistic standards. That kind of thinking simply puts you on the fast track to burnout and depression, which won't do you or your child any good. (Trust me on this one: I've been there.) So learn to practice self-compassion, which means "treat[ing] ourselves with the same kindness, caring, and compassion we would show to a good friend, or even a stranger for that matter," according to psychologist Kristin Neff, author of *Self-Compassion: Stop Beating Yourself Up and Leave Insecurity Behind*, one of my all-time favorite books.

## Work off Stress, Have Fun

As the parent of a child who is struggling with mental health or development problems, you may have to make a conscious decision to shift out of what one mother describes as "survival mode." Mary, mother of Janine (who has a mild intellectual disability and is on the autism spectrum) and Fiona (who has been diagnosed with bipolar disorder), explains: "For years, I was in survival mode and, unfortunately, that included not eating that well and gaining a lot of weight. I did not beat myself up about it, because I knew it was a coping mechanism and my focus was on the health and welfare of the children. When my third and youngest child was about three, I decided that I wanted to try to get into better shape. I started to get up very early to exercise. I have kept this up for over a decade. At one point I used to get up at 4 A.M. and run. Now I go to a local gym every morning at a more reasonable hour (6 A.M.). I still find myself seeking solace in carbs, but I feel better about myself. Exercise has been a good stress release."

Marie, mother of David, has found a soul-nourishing combo in yoga and cycling: "I started a yoga practice three times a week. I also cycle to work a few times a week."

Doing something creative is what keeps Laura going. Her son, Gabriel, has been diagnosed with Asperger syndrome (now simply referred to as autism spectrum disorder) and is currently being assessed for OCD. "I like to spend a bit of time each day doing something creative," she explains. "This helps keep me balanced. When we have a crazy-busy week and I don't get to do these things, I really start to feel the imbalance." Her advice to other parents? "It's easy to put yourself on the back burner, but you'll be a better parent (and person) if you take the time to look after yourself."

## Stay Connected

Andrew, father of David, has relied on a number of different strategies over the years to try to make life better for himself, his wife, and their other children, despite the worry and heartache associated with David's schizophrenia. He explains: "We tried to keep our work and family lives going as much as possible. We tried to tend to our other children's needs as best we could. We preserved our routines at home as much as possible. We sought help through our social circle. I got support from my colleagues at the time, who are social workers. My wife and I sought out a kindly psychiatrist, who saw us as a couple to work on the challenges of maintaining an ongoing connection with David. We also attended a weekly parent support group, which lasted a few months. And we attended as many appointments with David as we could to work with the professionals who were seeing him at the time. Both of us sought out ways to stay physically fit with regular exercise. One thing we got into more was dancing together to good old rock 'n' roll in our sunroom. That lifted our spirits at times. I play guitar and continued my playing alone or with a band I've been in for many years. We attend a vibrant church community on a fairly regular basis with many friends there. We knew people were praying for us. We resisted the urge to isolate or pull back at times. We keep trying to reach out and stay connected as best we can to family and friends. I've shared our story with a few people at work when it comes up. All of this connection and activity has helped us keep the awfulness of David's illness from overtaking our lives, individually and as a family. It has given us recreation, fun, and joy along with a sense of being cared for."

That may be a goal you feel you can set for yourself right now, during these wrenching and wretched early days—to keep the awfulness of your child's illness from overtaking your life, leaving room for hope and peace to take root. And if you feel like you might lose sight of this goal, ask a friend to remind you— or even take you—to do something for just 5 minutes a day that doesn't involve your child, so that you can focus, however briefly, on nurturing yourself.

Finding help for your child and working through his problems is more like a marathon than a sprint, and it will be run on a route with lots of loops and curves and hills and valleys. The one thing you know is that you have left the starting gate now and made your first positive progress. But you are in it for the long haul, so don't wait for your child's problems to be resolved before you start living the life you want. Start living it right now, accepting what is while striving for what is *possible*.

> When my parents were still able to, I used to have them come and help with the kids so I could escape with a girlfriend for a few days. It was heaven. The memories still sustain me. But my parents' health is failing and I haven't been able to get away for the last 5 years. Exercise is key for me, and so is having a purpose other than being a parent and running around to school and medical appointments. For me, that purpose is working in a field that allows me to help others.
>
> **Mary, mother of Janine, who has a mild intellectual disability and is on the autism spectrum, and Fiona, who has been diagnosed with bipolar disorder**

# 2

# Obtaining a Diagnosis

If only the process of diagnosing mental illness were as straightforward as diagnosing a garden-variety childhood illness. You'd take your child to the doctor's office, your doctor would examine your child, and you'd walk out with the name of an illness and a game plan for treating it.

Even the process of making the initial diagnosis is a lot more complicated—and a lot more time-consuming.

For one thing, the symptoms of psychiatric disorders in children are different from the symptoms in adults, because children are developmentally different from adults—and because children are constantly changing (which means their symptoms change along with them). A toddler who is experiencing anxiety may have trouble sleeping or eating. A school-age child who is experiencing anxiety may start acting up at school. And a teenager who is exhibiting anxiety may engage in self-harm, like cutting. Sometimes symptoms worsen. Sometimes symptoms improve. Sometimes they disappear altogether. Because no one has a crystal ball that can tell you which will be the case for your child, it makes sense to seek help for your child while holding on to your sense of hope and optimism that things will get better someday.

> A diagnosis is not an end point: it's a gateway to understanding how to map out the next part of the journey.
>
> **Leigh, mother of Skyler, who has been diagnosed with ADHD, anxiety, and depression**

Then there's the fact that children are less likely than adults to talk about what they are feeling. If a teenager is talking to anyone about what

28

she is experiencing, odds are that person is a friend and not a parent. What this means is that you are more likely to discover that your child is struggling by noticing a change in your child's behavior or an increase in physical complaints like headaches and stomachaches, than via a conversation in which your child explicitly asks for help. Your child's teachers may have noticed changes in your child too. They, along with other adults who know your child well, can be very helpful in providing information that is useful in making an accurate diagnosis.

Add to this the fact that it can take a long time to get an appointment with a child psychiatrist or child psychologist and the fact that you may have to jump through hoops with your insurance company or Medicaid to ensure that your child has access to and coverage for the right treatment, and you can see why waiting for diagnosis and treatment has become a rite of passage for so many—too many—children.

## Beginning Your Quest for Answers: The Doctor

Your child's pediatrician (or other primary care provider) can conduct a thorough examination of your child, ruling out any physical causes that could be contributing to his mental, emotional, or behavioral difficulties.

Depending on the results of those tests, the pediatrician might decide to conduct an assessment himself or refer your child to a specialist for a more comprehensive assessment. Depending on where you live and what resources are available in your area or via telemedicine, you might be referred to a children's mental health clinic, a child psychiatrist, or a child psychologist. The assessment process may include:

- Interviews with you and your child.
- Detailed questionnaires dealing with your child's medical history, developmental history, and behavior (to be completed by you, your child's other parent, and your child's teacher).
- A history of any physical or psychological traumas (a natural disaster, a death in the family—including the death of a beloved pet, adoption, abuse, and high levels of family conflict).
- A family history of mental, neurodevelopmental, and behavioral disorders.
- A review of reports from your child's school.
- Psychological testing for your child.

You might also wish to write a separate letter outlining your concerns. Writing a letter gives you the opportunity to describe specific concerns or to document specific behavioral incidents at home or at school that a generic questionnaire might not otherwise capture. The more specific you can be about describing your child's behavior, the more helpful it will be to the doctor or psychologist who is making the diagnosis and recommending treatment for your child.

Sometimes it can feel as though the assessment process focuses more on weaknesses than on strengths. You can help to balance things out by providing additional information that emphasizes your child's strengths to the person who is conducting the assessment. If you're not sure how to get started, try answering the following questions:

- What are your child's greatest strengths?
- What does your child really like about herself?
- Who does she turn to for support?
- What are your family's greatest strengths?
- Who does your family turn to for support?
- What supports have been the most helpful to your family and to your child?
- What types of supports do you wish had been available to your family and your child (or would you like to have available to your family and your child)?
- What have past experiences taught you about your child's and your family's ability to cope with challenging situations?
- In what positive ways have your child and your family changed as a result of these experiences?

In most cases, the information you are providing will be welcomed by the person conducting the assessment. In rare cases, it may be rejected or ignored. If the person conducting the assessment does not welcome this type of input, you might want to ask why. After all, you have invaluable insights to share about your child.

## Beginning Your Quest for Answers: The School

If your child is having difficulty functioning at school, the school is likely to recommend that an individualized education program (IEP) be developed to spell out the services and supports your child needs to be successful at school. If the school does not make this suggestion, but you feel that such support is warranted, you can request that your child undergo a comprehensive psychoeducational assessment (personality tests as well as assessments of academic skills and intelligence). Or, if you prefer, you can arrange for a psychologist in private practice to assess your child and then provide the school with the results of that assessment. Just be aware that the fees can be considerable—and that they can vary a lot, depending on where you live and the type and scope of the assessment. You could find yourself paying anywhere from a few hundred dollars to a few thousand dollars, so you'll want to be clear about the costs up front. Either way, assuming that your child is found to be eligible for support, the results of this assessment will be used to create an IEP—a legal document that guarantees your child the right to certain supports within the school system. "Remember that whatever individual education plan for your child you collaboratively establish with the school and sign off on is a legal document, and the school can be held to account if they are not holding up their side of the agreement," says Mark, whose son, Dawson, has been diagnosed with reactive attachment disorder, anxiety disorder, and moderate developmental disability. "Every child has the right to an education." See Chapter 10 for more about advocating for your child at school and your child's rights under such key pieces of legislation as the Individuals with Disabilities Education Act (IDEA), the Americans with Disabilities Act (ADA), and Section 504 of the Rehabilitation Act (which mandates the creation of so-called 504 plans for children whose disabilities "substantially" limit their ability to participate in school).

While you're touching base with your child's school, ask if any changes can be made to your child's environment right away while you're waiting for a formal assessment to be completed. Discuss your concerns and listen to the teacher's concerns. Keep the focus of your discussion on what would be of benefit to your child right now. Perhaps the school would be willing to consider reduced homework, modified start and end times to the school day, and helping your child access in-school supports such as counseling. Perhaps the teacher would consider changing your child's seat in the classroom so that he doesn't have to contend with as many distractions or providing him with strategies for working off the excess energy that is interfering with his learning. (See Chapter 7 for more about co-regulation and self-regulation.) It is important to know that, under federal law (two federal laws, actually: the Individuals with Disabilities Education Act and the Rehabilitation Act), your child has the right to a free appropriate public education (FAPE)—and one that provides the least restrictive environment possible for your child. In other words, it's not okay for schools to routinely siphon off students who are struggling and to sequester them in segregated classrooms, away from their peers. Schools should aim for inclusion whenever possible. (See Chapters 10 and 14 for more about the rights of individuals with disabilities.)

Of course, sometimes school simply isn't the best option for a particular child at a particular time. If you feel your child can't cope with attending school right now, ask the school what supports it can offer to your child while she continues her studies from home (access to a tutor, for example).

## If You're Dealing with a Crisis Situation

If your child is in crisis and you need her to be seen by someone right away, you can either take her to your local hospital emergency room (ideally a hospital with a pediatric emergency room) or call 911 for emergency assistance from police (if the situation is too dangerous for you to handle on your own or your child is at risk of harming herself or others). Here's what you need to know about these two options.

### Going to the Emergency Room

If you take your child to the emergency room when he is in crisis, he will initially be assessed by an intake doctor. Depending on what is revealed during the assessment (for example, whether your child is in imminent danger of harming himself or others), your child could be admitted to the hospital (assuming the hospital has a pediatric psychiatric unit), transferred to another hospital (which may mean that your child spends a day or two in the emergency ward while a social worker makes calls to other hospitals in the region to find him a suitable bed), or released back into your care with plans for follow-up.

> The decision to hospitalize a child is excruciatingly difficult. Once you start the process rolling, it can't be stopped. The system is not predictable. You might witness your child being restrained or medicated against his will, which is traumatizing to watch. The more you know about the process going in, the better, as it's important to know how to be your child's and your own, advocate.
>
> **Rashida, mother of Elijah, who has been diagnosed with bipolar disorder**

Depending on where you live, you may find that child psychiatric care is extremely difficult to access, even if your child is in crisis. Cheyenne recalls her family's experience: "Keisha was 11 the night we tried to have her admitted to a psychiatric hospital. They wouldn't take her because [according to them] her mental health crisis wasn't bad enough—this despite the fact that I had bruises up my entire arm and she had tried to kill my dog."

Regardless of whether your child is admitted to the hospital or released into your care, it is important to understand your treatment options, make informed decisions about your child's care, and ensure that there is some sort of care plan in place by the time you walk out the door, even if it's something as basic as a referral or a follow-up appointment. You don't want your child to fall through the cracks because one part of the system doesn't do a good enough job of talking to another.

## Calling 911

It is a terrifying thing to have to call the police because your child is in crisis, says Rashida. And she should know. "We had four huge police-men come into our house, grab our son, and handcuff him in our living room. It was very traumatic." It's not a decision that parents like Rashida make lightly—but sometimes there simply isn't any alternative. "We were exhausted. We would be the ones holding him for hours while he struggled and had tantrums," she recalls.

As Rashida's experience demonstrates, families are most likely to call 911 for assistance when a family member is in crisis: demonstrating intent to harm herself; exhibiting an immediate risk of suicide; behaving in a strange, unusual, or disorganized way; or becoming violent.

If you call 911, it is important to remain calm and explain to the opera-tor that your child is experiencing a mental health crisis and needs to go to the hospital to seek medical help. Describe what your child is doing and saying. When the police arrive, provide them with an up-to-date copy of your child's medical information (see the box below).

Understand that you won't be able to control the way police interact with your child once they arrive on the scene. You can hope that the offi-cers in question have received appropriate crisis intervention training (to equip them with the skills needed to deescalate conflicts involving people in distress) and that they will seek to provide your child with access to mental health services and supports rather than an express trip to the local jail, but, ultimately, the situation will be entirely in their hands. That's why

---

### Medical Information to Have Available on Your Child

- Contact information for your child's doctor.
- Highlights of your child's medical history.
- A list of medications currently being taken and, if applicable, psychiatric medications taken in the past, along with a brief note about the results of those medication attempts, including side effects.
- Your best advice to anyone trying to deal with your child.

many parents who feel they are likely to have to make that fateful 911 call at some point down the road choose to make contact with their local police force *before* their child is in crisis. "You have to have relationships with law enforcement, and you need to have a safety plan in place," says Liza Long, author of *The Price of Silence,* and mother of a teenager who has been diagnosed with bipolar disorder.

 **NOTE:** Be sure to note the names and badge numbers of police officers who respond to your call for your records and to jot down the date and time of their arrival.

Part of making a safety plan is being clear in your own head about the types of circumstances that would cause you to call the police. "A key question to think about is 'What is your own personal limit?'" says Rashida.

And, if you do have to make that call, remind yourself that you are doing this out of care and concern for your child and try to take solace in the fact that seeking emergency assistance could potentially help to turn an impossible situation around. That's how things played out for Rashida's family. Her son, Elijah, spent the next 6 months in the hospital, which gave doctors an opportunity to fine-tune his meds and help him work on his coping skills. "We hesitated to call for many years. Looking back, it probably would have been helpful to do it earlier."

> Our local police were very helpful when we needed assistance in getting Sam to the hospital for an involuntary hospitalization. We called our local precinct, explained the situation, and asked them to come to our home (without flashing lights or sirens) to encourage Sam to get in our car to go to the hospital, and it worked.
>
> **Linda, mother of Sam, who has been diagnosed with ADHD and learning disabilities**

## The Truth about Labels

Some parents are initially afraid to seek a diagnosis for their child, out of fear of what receiving "a label" might mean for their child.

Alison remembers the concerns she grappled with prior to seeking a diagnosis for her daughter, Charlotte, who has been diagnosed with an anxiety disorder: "I waited, because I was concerned that taking Charlotte to a professional would highlight her problems in her own mind and make things worse. I didn't want her to think of herself as a 'sick kid.' So I put it off until it was clear anxiety was interfering with some things that gave her pleasure. I don't think that ended up happening, though: I don't think she ended up seeing herself as a 'sick kid.'"

Leigh remembers experiencing similar feelings prior to seeking a diagnosis for her son, Skyler, who has been diagnosed with ADHD, anxiety, and depression: "I worried that if Skyler knew he was 'depressed' and 'anxious,' it might be a label he felt he had to carry always. I want him to be happy and not identify as being just the unhappy child."

Laura, whose son Gabriel has been diagnosed with Asperger syndrome and exhibits a lot of OCD-type behaviors, was concerned that other people might not be willing or able to look beyond any diagnostic "label" her son received. Fortunately, for the most part, she says, that hasn't proven to be the case.

"I was a bit worried that 'labeling' Gabriel would do more harm than good. I am completely over that, though. I have only ever had one conversation with someone who was blathering on about how people hide behind diagnoses rather than just discipline our kids—and how we all just want to feed our kids drugs so we don't have to deal with them. And I'm confident enough in my parenting now that I just ignored the person. I fear that younger, less experienced mothers might take that sort of nonsense to heart, though.

"Most adults have always liked Gabriel because he is very polite and well behaved, and the diagnoses just bought him more patience. For those adults who don't 'get' it (and those are becoming fewer and farther between), it just confirms their fears. There is still the odd person who acts as if autism is contagious: they can't get away from Gabriel fast enough. They tend to be ignorant, ill-informed adults, as a rule—and several of them are in my extended family.

"The same is true for kids. Gabriel has a few friends who are great, caring, sensitive children. Then there are a lot of kids who aren't necessarily his friends, but who treat him well because they know he has Asperger's. Then there are the few who are unkind (he's had two instances of bullying in his life), and they, like the adults, are just ill-informed, ignorant bigots."

Mara has found that being able to turn to a diagnosis to explain her son Jake's behavior has encouraged people to be more accepting of his differences. "People are kinder to my son now that I can explain to them that he did this or that because of his ADHD and that's just how it is. I'm glad that they are more accepting, but I wish people would be more accepting of uniqueness without requiring an explanation."

Mary explains, "Instead of standing there blankly listening to complete strangers in the shopping mall lecture me about controlling my child while she was having a meltdown, I could finally say, 'She is autistic and this is what children with autism do sometimes.' At one point I was tempted to have business cards printed with an explanation."

She is quick to add, however, that her daughters are so much more than any label could possibly convey: "Both of my daughters are amazing, wonderful people. They are not defined by their disability."

Language is important here. Defining the person by the diagnosis ("Jeff is schizophrenic") is highly stigmatizing and limiting. It is better to leave the door open to possibility by using language reflecting the fact that the diagnosis is just one ingredient in the recipe for a particular person ("Jeff has schizophrenia"—just like he has blue eyes and brown hair).

## The Waiting Game

Once you have decided to seek a diagnosis and put the wheels in motion, you may be shocked—and frustrated—to discover just how long it can take to obtain an assessment for a child who is struggling.

"Finding a psychiatrist, especially one who works with children and adolescents, can be a major challenge," says Kristina, mother of 18-year-old Clare. "Wait times for an appointment can be outrageously long for new and established patients alike."

Christine had a similar experience trying to access care for her son, Will, who was ultimately diagnosed with severe ADHD and an anxiety disorder. "I feel the wait time from first suspecting an issue to diagnosis was far too long. For about a year, we were left with no idea what was going on and no idea what to do to help Will."

Mary can relate to those feelings. "The worst part was the waiting and sense of hopelessness," the mother of two recalls. (Her daughter Janine has a mild intellectual disability and is on the autism spectrum, and her daughter Fiona has been diagnosed with bipolar disorder.) "We were told by our doctor, while our children's names sat on lists for assessment, that priority only went to urgent cases, and urgent cases meant the child had succeeded in injuring himself or someone else very seriously. And some of the doctors and psychiatrists we dealt with did not have the expertise to identify what might be wrong."

Sometimes the assessment process is put on hold for other reasons. Doctors may encourage you to take a wait-and-see approach as opposed to digging deep for answers right away. "When you have a child who starts to show behavioral difficulties at age 4, there are a lot of possible explanations. You'll hear things from doctors like 'Wait it out' or 'Maybe it's indigestion.' Nobody's really willing to make a diagnosis at that point," says Rashida.

"The process is challenging. You want answers right away, but that isn't always possible when you're dealing with a young child."

And sometimes we're the ones who put the brakes on the assessment process—because it's easier to bury our heads in the sand and deny that there's a problem than to face the unknown: "Our own denial as parents is a major barrier to overcome on the path to diagnosis and treatment," says Kristina, whose daughter, Clare, has been diagnosed with bipolar disorder and generalized anxiety disorder as well as food sensitivities and irritable bowel syndrome. "No one wants in on this journey, and it's hard not to shut down those early suspicions and just refuse to deal with it."

Parents might feel less afraid of obtaining a diagnosis if they understood that knowledge is power and that a diagnosis is the first step to putting crucial supports in place for their child, says Mara, mother of Jake, who has been diagnosed with ADHD, and Samantha, who has been diagnosed with anxiety. "I think parents need to understand that a diagnosis is a gift. It means that you can help your child. It may be scary, but it's necessary and it's actually a good thing."

## What to Do While You Wait

You may feel as though your family has been left in limbo while you wait for an assessment—and that there's nothing you can do to help your child in the meantime. In fact, there *are* things you can do while you are waiting for answers and supports.

### Connect with Other Parents Who Are Facing the Same Challenges

Look for online or face-to-face parent support groups for parents who have a child with mental health challenges. Parent support groups can be a great source of information and support on everything from effective parenting to advocacy techniques to tapping into services and supports. (See Chapters 4 and 12 and visit the book website, *www.anndouglas.net*, for more about parent support groups.)

### Focus on Staying Connected to Your Child

Your relationship with your child is key. Ask your child what he needs and how you can help. Be encouraging and accepting. Have realistic expectations for your child. And, above all, find ways every day to show your child just how much you care. See Chapters 6 and 7 for specific techniques that encourage connection and minimize conflict.

### Learn How to Advocate for Your Child

Be your child's voice if she is not able to speak for herself. Be as specific as possible in describing the worrisome changes that you are seeing in your child: a deterioration in functioning at home (difficulties with sleeping, eating, relationships, or behavior, poorer hygiene or reduced self-care, evidence of drug or alcohol use or early sexual activity); at school (academic or social difficulties, skipping school); or in the community (loss of interest in activities your child normally loves, conflict with the law, risk-taking behaviors). When you are advocating for your child, ask for the most appropriate care (based on the best evidence available and your understanding of your child's needs) as opposed to merely accepting what is being offered. Let your child's teacher know what specific classroom strategies would be helpful to your child. See Chapter 4 for additional tips on advocating for your child.

### Take the Best Possible Care of Yourself and Other Members of Your Family

Your child needs his family to remain healthy and strong. Try to line up support for yourself and other family members. Families need to be cared for too, after all. Research has demonstrated, in fact, that when parents are cared for, kids do better; and when kids are cared for, parents do better. While you're waiting to tap into support from outside the family, work at maximizing good health at home. See Chapters 5 and 9 for advice on stress management and leading a healthy lifestyle.

## You Have the Diagnosis: Now What?

You've paid attention to your parent radar, and you've taken the steps necessary to gather information about your child and seek an assessment. At last, you have a diagnosis that explains something about your child's condition. This is a very valuable, very helpful piece of the puzzle, but it's probably not going to be "the answer"—an all-encompassing explanation that allows you to make sense of everything your child has been experiencing.

A diagnosis is likely to result in more questions than answers—at least initially. Some of the questions you'll want to ask include:

- "What is this diagnosis likely to mean in terms of my child's daily life, both now and in the future?"
- "What can I do to help my child get well?"
- "What can I do to help my child cope with and manage these symptoms?"
- "Where can I turn for additional information and support?"

"Realize that diagnosing mental health issues, especially in children, is a complex exercise in educated guesswork," says Andrew, father of David. "There is no definitive test to make this an objective or scientific endeavor. It is more of an art based on a certain knowledge base that, at this point, is still somewhat limited, unfortunately."

And it's not unusual for an initial diagnosis to be tentative—or for a child to receive a series of diagnoses (and treatment recommendations) that evolve over time.

"It has been over 3 years, and I still don't have a mental health diagnosis that I can be sure of," says Rebecca, whose daughter, Madalyn, has been diagnosed with learning disabilities and seems to exhibit some of the characteristics of ODD, sensory integration disorder, and ADHD. "We have been involved with one children's mental health agency for about 2 years and have seen an expert psychiatrist at another (his advice was 'wait and see'), but no one seems interested in diagnosing. And, of course, without a diagnosis, there aren't any guaranteed supports or accommodations."

"We're still working on a diagnosis," says Lisa. "We started when Laura was 4. We saw one child development specialist after 1 year, but she couldn't help without a definitive medical diagnosis. We saw the pediatrician, who gave a preliminary diagnosis of OCD and anxiety, possibly FASD [fetal alcohol spectrum disorder]. Laura is borderline ADHD, which mirrors FASD. We got in the queue for an FASD assessment. After 18 months, she was assessed at age 6, and there was enough evidence to refer her for a more comprehensive assessment. We're still waiting."

Karen's experience was even more discouraging: "Spencer's official diagnosis of PDD-NOS [recently renamed an autism spectrum disorder when the American Psychiatric Association updated its diagnostic manual] came 9 years after I first became aware that there was an issue," she recalls. "There were many interim diagnoses and lots of dead-end roads. He was given temporary 'labels' such as schizophrenic, oppositional defiant disorder, and just plain old spoiled."

Andrew appreciates the fact that the experts went to great lengths to decide on the right diagnosis for David, even if the process was painstakingly long. "Several diagnoses were made over time, including ADHD as a child, mood disorder in early adolescence, oppositional defiant disorder, drug-induced psychosis, and finally—at around age 17—schizophrenia became and remains the working diagnosis," he recalls. "We appreciate the fact that a diagnosis in David's case was complicated and could only be made over time as more information was forthcoming in terms of his symptoms and behavior. We felt the professionals all did a good job in being careful not to jump to conclusions too early."

> By the time we knew David most likely had schizophrenia, we had gone through a long period of anxiety and stress. Finding out he had this terrible illness was almost anticlimactic. It had been running through our minds as a distinct possibility for some time prior to the formal diagnosis being made. I think we had been in a grieving process all along, realizing he was drifting out to sea and that there wasn't a lot we could do about it. We felt helpless, anxious, sad, and angry at various times and sometimes all at once.
> **Andrew, father of David, who has been diagnosed with schizophrenia**

## What If You Don't Agree with the Diagnosis?

If you feel that the current diagnosis for your child does not accurately represent his behavior, it is important to raise your concerns. After all, you know your child best, and the more accurate your child's diagnosis is, the more likely your child is to receive the treatments and supports he needs to thrive. Don't be intimidated by the fact that members of your child's treatment team have specialized knowledge about your child's disorder. You are bringing specialized expertise to the table as well: in-depth knowledge about your child.

So be prepared to speak up and advocate for your child until he receives an accurate diagnosis. "Trust your gut if you feel that a diagnosis is not on par with what you believe is the issue," says Jodi, whose son, Kyle, has been diagnosed with Asperger syndrome, a learning disability, generalized anxiety disorder, and ADHD. "Keep pushing until you find the right clinician and come to a conclusion that makes sense based on what you are seeing with your child."

## Talking with Your Child about the Diagnosis

Of course, one of the most important conversations you'll have about your child's diagnosis is the conversation you'll have with your child. During this conversation, you'll want to explain to your child, in practical terms, exactly what the diagnosis means.

Young children may focus on the physical symptoms they've been experiencing, like stomachaches or headaches. They will need your help to make sense of—and learn to cope with—feelings that seem overwhelming or scary.

Teenagers may think they are weird, weak, or going crazy. They need to know that their thoughts, feelings, and actions make perfect sense, given what they've been experiencing, and that there are ways to make their life easier. They also need to know that you continue to love and accept them, that you will help them deal with these challenges, and that you will help them find and access the care they need. You'll want to encourage teens to play an active role in thinking about what types of supports would be most helpful to them in addressing their challenges and maximizing their mental health (as opposed to arbitrarily making such treatment decisions yourself). The more involved your child is in co-creating (with you and members of her mental health team) a treatment plan that meets her needs, the more likely she is to buy into that treatment plan—and the more confident and in control she will feel about the situation.

"We were very honest with both children about their mental health and their needs," says Mara. "We don't believe in mincing words or being dishonest with them. Their mental illnesses are part of who they are. It may not define them, but it's as much a part of them as their hair color."

When you're having this conversation, it's important to ensure that your child understands that a mental health diagnosis doesn't mean there's something wrong with her. It just means that she's differently wired—and this implies having unique strengths as well as facing unique challenges.

"Help kids to really understand their diagnosis and to see it as a difference, not a disability," advises Tara, whose son Aiden has been diagnosed with autism and ODD and whose son Owen has been diagnosed with anxiety and ADHD. "Acknowledge that things are different for them. Don't discount their pain. But help them not to be victims. Help them to see how amazing they are, and that autism or ADHD or whatever gives them advantages, too—that thinking differently than others is okay."

Your child also needs to know that the most difficult part of the journey the two of you are making together (the part when you don't know what you're dealing with and there aren't any supports in place) is already behind you. Things should get easier from this point onward (although you both still have a lot of hard work ahead of you).

Christine found that letting her son, Will, know that they were in this thing together—and that his struggles weren't anybody's fault—allowed them to move forward in a positive way. She explains: "Since diagnosis, our relationship has improved. We now have a known cause for the struggles Will was having, and a way to deal with them. He knows it's not his fault and I know it's not mine. His mental health issues have nothing to do with anything either of us have done wrong. My advice to other parents would be to embrace this knowledge and to move forward with a treatment plan as a team."

## How You May Be Feeling

Now that you finally have a diagnosis in your hands, you may be surprised to find yourself experiencing a mix of emotions.

"My primary emotion when Aiden was finally diagnosed was just pure relief. It had been such a long, hard road and finally someone was saying to me, 'Yes, there is a reason he acts this way, and no, it is not because you suck as a mother.' I actually wept with relief, holding that piece of paper in my hand," recalls Tara, mother of Aiden and Owen. "With Owen's diagnosis, I was really sad. Since I have dealt with anxiety and depression my whole life and my husband has ADD [attention deficit disorder], I so badly didn't want to pass that on. It hurt my heart that my child was feeling that same way, and it brought up all sorts of emotions from my own childhood."

Many parents are relieved to discover just how much their children's lives improve after a diagnosis. Their children gain new insights into their own behavior. And they gain access to services and supports that simply weren't available to them prediagnosis.

"The diagnosis improved David's life 100%," says Marie. "It was a gift to him. Before the diagnosis and treatment, David blamed himself much of the time. 'What is wrong with me?' he would say. He was often miserable and felt like he was failing. Once we were able to explain that his brain runs at a different speed than other people's . . . he felt vindicated. It wasn't that he was bad or stupid or anything; he just had a brain that was wired a bit differently."

"I wasn't the only one asking, 'What is wrong with my child?'" recalls Mary, mother of Janine and Fiona. "My girls knew they were different. They just didn't know why. The diagnoses helped them understand themselves a little better. Janine knows she is autistic, but she doesn't dwell on it. She is always moving forward, looking for a new life goal to achieve. And Fiona has a scientific mind. She researches her symptoms and the science around her bipolar disorder.

"The diagnoses also helped with 'the system'—getting accommodations through school and sometimes explaining to the police and other officials why one of the children behaved the way she did."

You may find that having some sort of explanation for your child's behavior allows you to be more compassionate toward your child—and yourself.

"The diagnosis helped us understand what was happening in David's head," says Marie. "It made it easier to relate to him, and we were less angry at him for getting distracted, forgetting things, and so on. We could concentrate on helping him overcome these challenges. It made things better at home."

Gabriel's mother, Laura, agrees: "Overall, a diagnosis has bought a certain degree of patience: it makes the odd behavior more acceptable, because it's 'a real thing.'"

Christine feels much better about her parenting abilities. "Before diagnosis, I often blamed myself for Will's issues. Perhaps I was too strict or not strict enough. Maybe I needed to improve his diet or take away the TV. After the diagnosis, I was able to recognize that none of Will's issues were a result of bad parenting. It was a huge relief."

Jodi experienced similar feelings of relief after her son Kyle's diagnosis: "We blamed ourselves before he was diagnosed. We thought we were just bad parents."

Many parents find themselves taking new approaches to parenting in the wake of their child's diagnosis. They become aware that one-size-fits-all parenting solutions won't work anymore (assuming they ever worked at all).

"We definitely are more sensitive to their needs," says Mara. "The diagnosis has made us understand, even more, that each child needs to be parented differently, according to his or her strengths and weaknesses." (See Chapter 6 for more about parenting strategies.)

Tara agrees: "Knowing Aiden had autism changed the way we parented. We were able to figure out so much more. We took classes. We researched. We knew what we were dealing with, finally."

Mary remembers the moment when she realized her approach to parenting needed to shift. "For me, the unknown was scarier than knowing what the problem was. I am a problem solver by nature. So tell me the diagnosis and I will research and adapt. If I don't know what is wrong, how do I know whether I am helping or harming my kids when I respond to them? For years, I dealt with problem behavior by trying to impose timeouts, counting to three, and all those other parenting techniques we are bombarded with. I frustrated myself and my kids. The techniques didn't work and they were never going to work. I felt like a failure.

"I remember sitting in a parking lot at an animal farm with Janine one day. She had had a tantrum and injured a family member. I kept saying, 'It's easy. Just say you're sorry, and we will go and have a nice day.' She didn't budge. I was looking for remorse and contrition from a child who couldn't control an impulse, didn't empathize, or feel remorse. Fiona, ever the wise one, said, 'Mommy, I don't think it's easy for her to say sorry.' She was right and we left the car and had a nice day."

## Confronting Stigma

Having a child with a psychiatric disorder puts you on the front lines of the battle against stigma. And the nature of your child's illness is likely to determine how hard and how often you have to fight that battle. While we've come a long way as a society when it comes to speaking openly about the debilitating effects of depression, we still have a long way to go when it comes to talking about many other types of disorders.

"The biggest challenge has been in dealing with people who don't believe mental illness exists," says Christine. "For example, just this week I've heard people saying that ADHD is merely the medicalization of being a brat. I'm mostly able to tune these people out, but I worry about how my child will deal with this type of attitude as he gets older. How will it make him feel about himself? Will it make him want to go off medication? Will he feel like there's something 'wrong' with him? That he's bad? This remains one of my biggest concerns."

Mara shares Christine's concerns about "the terrible prejudices against ADHD and the misconceptions surrounding it. . . . Imagine living your life thinking everyone believes you're faking or you could behave differently if you wanted to," she says.

Mara resents the fact that people think Jake's ADHD is "made up" or that "we can just discipline it out of him or love it out of him or something." People are "really weird" in the way they react to both ADHD and anxiety, she notes. "People say stupid things like 'What does a kid have to worry about?' or 'ADHD is overdiagnosed. He is just active.'"

Some parents deal with their concerns about stigmatization by choosing to share details of their child's diagnosis with selected people only.

"I only told teachers [about Charlotte's anxiety] if they needed to know for a specific reason," says Alison. "They've all been supportive."

"Because of the stigma associated with ADHD medications, we've only shared Will's diagnosis with close friends and family," adds Christine. "They haven't treated Will any differently."

Mara and her husband disagreed about how open to be with others about their children's diagnoses. "To him, a mental health issue is something to be kept private and secret. But I wanted to be open with people about it—particularly the ADHD. I didn't want my kids to feel stigmatized but rather to understand that their mental health issues are part of them (although not who they are)," she explains.

Jackie, whose two sons, David and John, have both been diagnosed with a psychotic disorder, says that she continues to find it difficult to speak openly about her sons' illnesses. "Stigma and all the loneliness and sadness that come with it scare me to death. I am getting better at admitting the kids have a mental health issue, but I am still unable to admit to the diagnosis. I'm not sure why. I want to say it is totally to protect my children's dignity, but to tell you the truth, it could be to save myself some embarrassment too. I think this will take some time to overcome."

"When it comes to schizophrenia, there is a great reluctance on the part of families to talk about it," says Marvin, whose son David has schizophrenia. He notes that some of the worst experiences of stigma that his family has encountered have been while dealing with people within the mental health care system itself. "A student doctor told my wife she did not know that anyone with schizophrenia could have a good outcome. A nurse on the psych ward, when my son was last in, told him that, with schizophrenia, he was stupid to think he could ever work or even do volunteer work. My son has worked with kids with special needs and is presently a volunteer."

Liza Long, author of *The Price of Silence* and mother of a teenager who has been diagnosed with bipolar disorder, shares Marvin's outrage about these types of encounters but believes that the tide is beginning to turn when it comes to stigma—in part because people are beginning to speak frankly and openly about their experiences: "We could have a tipping point at any time if people keep talking and advocating and demanding change."

## The Blame Game

The process of having your child diagnosed with a mental illness tends to be stressful. Not only do you have to take time off work to take your child to a series of appointments with mental health professionals, but you have to be prepared to speak openly about all aspects of your family's life. Sadly, it's not uncommon for parents to emerge from this process feeling blamed for their children's difficulties rather than supported in their efforts to obtain help for their child.

"I was completely horrified by the process of getting Aiden diagnosed," recalls Tara. "It was a nightmare from start to finish, filled with professionals basically making me feel like a horrible, awful parent and blaming me for everything he did, until I finally found someone who would actually listen. We lost years when we could have been working with him and accessing services that could have truly benefited him."

"When they assessed Samantha, they told me she had anxiety and that it was my fault because I'd overparented her," recalls Mara. "This was ridiculous, because I'm the opposite of an overparenter. So, my advice is, if anyone tells you it's your fault, go somewhere else for a real conversation about your child's mental health."

"I realize that having a child with mental health issues requires a very strong parent and adaptive parenting techniques, but we were growing very tired of hearing that it was always our fault. It seemed that people were quick to point the finger at the cause without offering any valid solutions," says Mark, father of Dawson.

"Overall, there's the feeling that whatever is wrong with the child is the fault of the parent, especially the mother," adds Rebecca.

So if you're feeling blamed, know that you're not the only one. A lot of people are quick to blame parents when a child is struggling, says Long: "There's still very much the sense that it's bad parenting, end of story."

Of course, the blame many parents feel directed at them by other people pales in comparison to the blame they pin on themselves.

"My husband and I have gone through times of blaming ourselves for both our children's issues," says Tara. "We are still working through it. Genetics are heartless. And we know we didn't do everything right with Aiden, since we had no idea what we were dealing with when he was little. We would have done so many things differently if we had known he had autism."

Rebecca understands those feelings. Still awaiting a mental health diagnosis for her daughter, Madalyn, she says, "I can't let go of thinking that this is my fault. Studies tell me that single parenting is at fault or genetics are at fault or poverty is at fault. I also feel very guilty about the postpartum depression I had when I was a brand-new mom and wonder whether a lack of attachment is to blame. I have no advice on how to cope with this other than to not read the studies and to be very dismissive of whatever the media is saying this week/month/year."

Laura has managed to sidestep the blame game herself but notes that her husband struggles with feelings of self-blame in the aftermath of their son's diagnosis "because the genetic component definitely comes from his side of the family." She doesn't consider trying to figure out the origins of a specific diagnosis particularly helpful, "except for the scientists who are doing research." She prefers to take an "onward and upward approach."

Mara has chosen to take the same approach in the aftermath of her two children's diagnoses. "Whatever I did before I knew something was wrong, well, I can't change that. I can only go forward and be the best parent possible for my child. Sure, I made a lot of mistakes, but I can't undo them. I can only be better now, do my research, and help my children to be their best selves, and set them up for success within and beyond their limitations."

Lily says she'll always be working through her daughter Asia's diagnosis with borderline personality disorder (BPD), but that, over time, a series of realizations she's reached have allowed her to accept the fact that she may have contributed to her daughter's difficulties through genes, environment, or both, and to accept that she did the best she could.

> The past is the past. Focus on making things better now, not eating yourself alive over what you might have done wrong.
> **Alison, mother of Charlotte, who has been diagnosed with an anxiety disorder**

"At some point, I think we all come to this place or someplace like it: I failed my children in many ways, and I'll never know what might have happened had I not done so. I loved them with all my heart and did the very best I could with the understanding and ability I had at the time. It is essential that I forgive myself in order to be the person I have the potential to be today and in the future. Mental illness is incredibly complex, and we will never know what mix of genetics and environmental factors contributed to my daughter's illness. I have to accept that and move on. Guessing is a waste of time and energy. I find comfort in the things I was able to do 'right': being an effective advocate, always being a loving mom no matter how awful things got, being there."

For Andrew, a key part of coming to terms with his son's illness was accepting the fact that parenting—even good parenting—is no guarantee that a child will be spared struggles. "My wife and I both work in the field of education and children's mental health, so we've been exposed to a lot of information, over the years, related to parenting. I taught parenting classes for several years in the past. This was both an advantage and a challenge," he explains. "We certainly had our times of doubting our parenting skills in the face of David's evolving and increasing challenges. However, the more we knew about schizophrenia, the more we understood that even if we had been super parents, it would not have made much difference in terms of the final outcome. Good-enough parenting is all most of us can hope for and, in most cases, it is adequate."

Parents who have children who are thriving as well as children who are struggling find it easier to keep the impact of parenting in perspective. They can see firsthand that it is possible to use the same parenting strategies with different kids and get different results. This doesn't mean we should minimize the importance of using the most effective parenting strategies we can: we simply need to recognize that parenting is just one of many factors that influence whether a particular child struggles or thrives.

Genetics, of course, is another.

Joanne felt a lot of guilt in the aftermath of her son William's depression diagnosis. "I have a long family history of mental illness and wondered if I had any right to have children at all. I started to feel as if I had ruined my son's life and grieved that he would suffer as I have." She had to work through these feelings before she was able to recognize that she had a lot to offer her son *because* of her own struggles with depression. "We can talk about life and challenges freely . . . I can coach him through the difficult times because he's not hiding anything from me. He knows I've been there and that I'm not judging him. He's able to ask for help from me and others, and that makes a huge difference."

Alison feels that her own hard-won insights into what it's like to live with anxiety have allowed her to be a better parent to Charlotte. "At least as a parent with anxiety, I 'get' her and know she needs help, not just discipline."

Rebecca has been motivated to advocate for her daughter, Madalyn, because she wants her daughter to receive mental health treatment early— the very type of help Rebecca would have benefited from during her own growing-up years. She explains: "I have had depression since I was a child. It started when I was about 9 and I'm 34 now. I've been on and off—mostly on—antidepressants since I was 18. So, Madalyn is not the only person in our home dealing with mental health issues. Madalyn's issues often trigger depression in me—or I'm less able to deal with them because of my depression. But, on the other hand, I've been more on top of dealing with her issues, because I don't want her mood issues to be ignored (as mine were as a child) and I want to get her the help she needs now."

## What You Can Do to Help Now

It's important to realize that a diagnosis, while important, has its limitations. It may help you understand what your child is dealing with and open the door to new treatment options, but it doesn't replace you as the biggest force for change in your child's life. You will still need to figure out what types of supports and accommodations are most suitable for your child, with help from the mental health professionals who end up working with your child. And you'll still need to advocate on your child's behalf to put these supports in place (see Chapter 4). You'll also need to work one on one with your child to motivate and inspire her to envision the possibility of recovery and to set goals for herself that will guide her along that path. (See

Chapter 13 for more about clinical recovery versus personal recovery: they aren't the same thing.)

Instead of thinking of a diagnosis and treatment as miracle cures that will save your child, think of them as tools that you and your child can use as he begins to map out the path to greater wellness, with a lot of love and support from you. And embrace the fact that while diagnoses may evolve and treatment plans may change, you are the constant in your child's life, which is why you have the potential to make all the difference for him.

So take whatever help is available and find a way to make it work for your child and your family, advises Lily. "A diagnosis of mental illness generally means that some help is available, and even if it is too little or not the right kind, the difference between help and no help is profound."

## How to Get Support

Of course, one of the best sources of support is the support you are able to receive from other parents who have weathered the storm. "You need to find allies in other parents who have that shared experience," insists Grace, whose son Alex has been diagnosed with Asperger syndrome (now referred to as autism spectrum disorder). "The professionals haven't necessarily walked in your shoes."

And one thing other parents can do is help you keep your child's diagnosis in perspective: "I remember someone told me, 'No matter what diagnosis your kid has, it's still the same kid you had before the diagnosis,'" says Sofia, whose 11-year-old daughter, Gabriela, has been diagnosed with ADHD and dyslexia.

Whether you connect with other parents via a formal support group (either online or face-to-face) or via your circle of friends, such support can make the difference between thriving and merely surviving as a parent of a child with a mental health, neurodevelopmental, or behavioral challenge. Parents who have walked the same path can help you decide what to ask for and how to ask for it when you're advocating on your child's behalf. They can celebrate successes and help you put setbacks in perspective. And they can remind you to take breaks from the hard work of parenting so that you will have something left to give your child tomorrow.

# 3

# Starting Treatment

Your child has received her diagnosis. The next logical step is treatment. And, as at every stage in this journey, there is a learning process for you and your family, and there are decisions that will need to be made. Much of this will be difficult, but remember, too, that you are not alone, and you can learn from the experience of parents who have made this journey before you.

## Making Decisions about Treatment

Before your child starts treatment, you should be given information about her assessment (a debriefing about the basic findings and an explanation of the diagnosis if a diagnosis was reached) and details about the recommended course of action for addressing problems identified during the assessment. Issues that might be raised in this discussion include goals for treatment (for example, improved relationships, fewer disruptive behaviors), the specific methods to be used to achieve these goals, and the proposed time frame for treatment. The types of treatments recommended might include therapy

> I've learned to trust my instincts. I actually know a lot, and I'm the best expert when it comes to my daughter. Social workers and psychiatrists might be experts in their field, but my child is unique, not just a diagnosis.
>
> **Rebecca, mother of Madalyn, who has been diagnosed with learning disabilities and seems to exhibit some of the characteristics of ODD, sensory integration disorder, and ADHD**

(individual, family, or group sessions), behavioral parent skills training (parenting courses designed to provide you with new skills and approaches for dealing with your child's behavior), and medication.

You should be given an opportunity to offer feedback on the plans for treatment. Not only can you offer unique insights into the suitability of various treatment approaches for your child (you know your child better than anyone else, after all), you'll also be able to let the clinician know whether the treatment goals make sense for your child and whether they are realistic for your child and your family.

You might also want to consider whether your child could have input into decisions about treatment (something that will be determined by his age, his ability, and his degree of wellness), whether your child is likely to cooperate with the treatments being proposed, whether you have strong feelings (pro or con) about any of the recommended treatments, and whether your family can commit to everything that is being suggested, given your current resources (both financial and time). Should certain elements of treatment be prioritized? What would be the pros and cons of phasing in various elements of treatment as opposed to tackling all elements at once? These are the types of issues that should be discussed up front, so that you don't have to experience the frustration of realizing, mid-process, that the treatment game plan isn't manageable for your child or your family.

You'll want to find out how and when your child's progress will be evaluated. If your child is struggling at school, you might want to consider including someone from the school in the treatment planning process—perhaps the special education teacher or your child's classroom teacher—so that this person can offer insights into what might be workable in that setting and then report back about your child's progress.

You'll also want to be clear about what role you as a family will be expected to play. For example, will you be expected to provide information about your child's behaviors (in a behind-the-scenes consulting role), support the efforts of your child's therapist (by helping your child participate in the treatment process and work at home on the skills he is acquiring through therapy, and by sharing treatment strategies with your child's school), or be involved in treatment sessions (by attending your child's individual treatment sessions with him and participating in family therapy)?

It is important to ask questions about all aspects of treatment so that you can make an informed decision about proceeding. These might include:

- "What are my child's and my family's treatment options?"
- "What types of studies have been done to demonstrate the effectiveness of these treatments with children with the same disorder as my child?" (What you're looking for is reassurance that the treatments

being recommended reflect the best evidence about what has been *proven* to work, as opposed to someone's best guess about what *might* work.)

- "What are the risks and benefits of the various treatment options?"
- "What is the likelihood of the various treatments helping my child and my family?"

Don't just focus on the treatment options that are being recommended. You'll also want to consider what other types of approaches to treatment might benefit your child, given what you know about your child and her disorder. As Stephanie puts it: "Informed choice means understanding all the options."

And sometimes it means doing some out-of-the-box thinking about the types of treatments and supports that would be most helpful to your child right now. "You have to just keep rearranging the puzzle pieces," says Jennifer, whose daughter, Jessica, experiences a variety of physical and mental health difficulties related to her tuberous sclerosis diagnosis. "I called a brain trauma rehab center in the nearest big city (because Jessica's situation is much more like brain trauma than autism or anything like that), and they had just hired a neuropsychologist with experience treating adolescents with brain injuries. She was exactly the right person. Interestingly, she ended up having more sessions with Jess's dad and me than with Jess, basically training us in how to cope! And she was very focused on what Jess wanted and what Jess's goals were. Almost no one else has ever focused on that."

> Clare didn't start OT until nearly 2 years after her diagnosis. Not one of the various health care providers she saw during that time suggested it as a useful intervention. I only thought of it myself when I was watching the *Parenthood* television series. One of the characters on that show has Asperger's, and there is a storyline showing some of the services she was provided. It occurred to me that some of the techniques might be helpful for Clare. I sought out a practice in our community, and it's been an extremely productive element of Clare's overall care plan for the past 6 months. During her intake with the OT facility, they asked how I'd heard about them and why I was considering OT, and when I told them, they laughed and said that television show is currently their #1 referrer.
>
> **Kristina, mother of 18-year-old Clare, who has been diagnosed**
> **with bipolar disorder and generalized anxiety disorder**
> **and also suffers from food sensitivities and irritable bowel syndrome**

Consider this, though: if an exciting new treatment sounds too good to be true, it probably is. And while you might think you have nothing to lose by trying an experimental treatment with your child, you might be overlooking the cost of wasted time. As the Child Mind Institute notes on its website: "Time spent exploring non-evidence-based care may seem like a good investment, but it comes with an 'opportunity cost' to your child. That is, the longer kids miss out on treatment that really affects symptoms, the more time they'll spend impaired and, in many cases, missing out on crucial learning and development that goes on during childhood and adolescence. Their disorder may also grow worse without intervention." It's also important to recognize that herbal remedies aren't without side effects, and they can be dangerous when combined with other medications.

You might want to inquire about the qualifications of the people your child will be working with: what types of training they have received, how long they have been working in the field of children's mental health, whether they are licensed through any professional organizations that require clinical practitioners to adhere to a particular code of practice or code of ethics. And you'll definitely want to find out what your child can expect from the treatment sessions themselves: the type of therapy offered, the length and format of a typical session, the frequency of appointments, the number of sessions, and the expected outcomes. "It's difficult to know which treatments to pursue or how long to stick with them, particularly when you're driving long distances and/or paying out of pocket," says Eve, the mother of three daughters who have all dealt with adoption-related trauma and behavioral issues. Sofia, whose 11-year-old daughter, Gabriela, has been diagnosed with ADHD and dyslexia, agrees: "You can spend a fortune on things that don't even work." So be sure to find out up front whether you have to pay out of your own pocket to access any of these services, particularly alternative or experimental treatments that may not yet be covered by your insurance company.

So now you know which types of treatments and supports are most likely to be helpful for your child. How quickly can you expect treatment to begin? The answer to that question is a gigantic "It depends." How quickly treatment begins is likely to be determined by the nature of your child's diagnosis (the "seriousness" of your child's mental health or development challenge) and by the number of children in your area seeking access to treatment.

The patchwork-quilt nature of our mental health system—we don't have a single integrated system that delivers care—means that bureaucratic glitches can and do occur. Referrals get lost. Names fall off waiting lists.

And children and their parents end up paying the price. (See Chapter 14 for more on how the system could be improved to better meet the needs of children, youth, and families.)

It can be more than a little disheartening to discover that you have to try to chase down a referral that went astray. But, like it or not, this task falls to you as your child's parent. "So much depends on you," says Jennifer. "It is so hard and scary. You just have to go and go and go."

"It is important to stay on top of the process all the time," adds Sarah, whose daughter, Veronica, has been diagnosed with Asperger syndrome (now considered simply an autism spectrum disorder) and anxiety. She is the first to admit that this can be a time-consuming and exhausting task. "First, you have to figure out what you are entitled to, which is not easy. Then you have to figure out how to be persistent without looking like a crazy person or a stalker. Not everyone has the time or the resources to get through this."

## What's on the Therapy Menu?

To make the best possible treatment decisions for your child, it's important to understand what types of therapy are available. That way, you can consider what's being offered to your child and your family and what other types of therapy options may be available to your child. Depending on your family's circumstances, you may be able to arrange to provide your child with access to additional supports, including therapeutic recreational programs, on your own.

More than one *type of therapy* may be recommended for your child (for example, cognitive-behavioral therapy [CBT] plus behavioral activation treatment), with such therapy being delivered either by the same therapist or by different therapists. (Imagine different layers of therapy being applied at the same time or on different occasions—kind of like mental health sunscreen.) And depending on your child and family's needs, different *approaches to therapy* may be recommended as well: individual (your child and his therapist), family (your family, your child, and your therapist), and/or group therapy (your child, his peers, and a therapist).

In addition to considering your specific treatment options, you'll want to consider whether your child and your family are able to forge an emotional connection with the clinician who will be delivering the therapy. A positive therapeutic relationship—one based on genuine warmth and acceptance, in which you and your child are treated with kindness and respect—can make all the difference for your child and your family.

The list below is by no means complete, but it does include the most common types of therapies currently available to children and adolescents with mental health challenges. Directly under the heading for each treatment, I've listed problems it's been demonstrated to help treat, just to make it easy for you to find the treatments you might be interested in. *Keep in mind, however, that the conditions listed for each type of therapy are only examples; these lists are not comprehensive or all-inclusive.* You'll find some additional types of therapy and other related interventions (occupational therapy, psychosocial education for parents) described in the glossary at the back of the book (see Appendix A).

## Cognitive-Behavioral Therapy (CBT)

**Proven effective for depression, anxiety, OCD, eating disorders, PTSD, schizophrenia, some specific problems associated with psychosis, and for dealing with issues related to social skills problems**

CBT is based on the idea that our thoughts, feelings, and behaviors are all interconnected and that changing our thinking can result in changes to our feelings and our behavior (just as changing our behavior can change the way we think and feel). At a biological level, CBT helps to tame the amygdala, which can get caught up in endless loops of what-if thinking, by focusing on more rational thinking processes, which activate the parts of the brain involved in logic and reason.

CBT tends to focus on:

- Problem-solving training: for example, helping children who are prone to aggression ask themselves if it is possible they are misinterpreting the intentions of others as hostile.
- Cognitive restructuring: helping children identify unhelpful beliefs that may be making their lives more difficult—and ways that thinking differently could lead to feeling differently.
- Emotional literacy: helping children recognize that emotions can be changed and that we can take control of our emotions by learning how to recognize the early warning signs of rising emotion, and helping them understand that the inner dialogue we have with ourselves has the power to increase or decrease the intensity of our emotions.
- Relaxation training: teaching children to use relaxation techniques as a coping tool. Depending on your child's age and the specific treatment goals that are being pursued, your child's therapist may

use games, role playing, charades, art activities, board games, or puppets to work on some of these skills.

CBT has been proven effective in treating a variety of problems, including depression, anxiety, OCD, eating disorders, PTSD, and schizophrenia. CBT has also been demonstrated to improve symptoms like delusions, distress, and anxiety in people experiencing psychosis. Researchers from the Institute of Psychiatry at King's College London discovered that the parts of the brain that are activated in times of threat become less reactive in people who have participated in CBT. What's more, a small pilot study conducted by the same group of researchers found that CBT is effective in reducing symptoms of insomnia and the feelings of paranoia that often accompany sleep deprivation in people with psychosis.

CBT is proving to be a promising treatment for addressing symptoms of anxiety in very young children (ages 3 to 7). It is already a well-established technique for addressing anxiety in children 8 years and older.

## Dialectical Behavior Therapy (DBT)

**Proven effective for BPD, eating disorders, depression, substance abuse, suicidal and self-injuring behaviors, and emotional regulation**

DBT builds on the principles of CBT but also focuses on teaching mindfulness (living in the present moment with awareness and acceptance), emotional regulation, distress tolerance, and interpersonal skills through both individual and group therapy. The word *dialectical* suggests getting to the truth by arguing from contradictory points of view, and DBT involves learning how to hold two seemingly contradictory ideas in your mind at the same time, for example, accepting yourself as you are right now while also committing to work to change yourself.

DBT was originally designed as a treatment for BPD in women with a history of suicidal tendencies. It has since been adapted to treat other conditions, including eating disorders, depression, substance abuse, and suicidal and self-injuring behaviors. It is particularly helpful for adolescents who are having difficulty regulating emotions and behaviors, experiencing chaotic relationships with peers and adults, or experiencing a feeling of emptiness. DBT is typically offered to teenagers as opposed to younger children, but a recent study has highlighted its usefulness for younger children, too.

Some families have had tremendous success with DBT. "It was dialectical behavior therapy that finally turned things around, helping my daughter develop tolerance to negative emotions and challenges in her life, manage her emotions and her thoughts through mindfulness, develop coping strategies, and come to accept her emotions," says Lily, whose daughter, Asia, has been diagnosed with BPD.

## Acceptance and Commitment Therapy (ACT)

**Proven effective for anxiety, depression, OCD, self-harm, substance abuse, psychosis**

ACT encourages individuals to live their lives consciously and in accordance with their values. It emphasizes acceptance, mindfulness, and behavioral change. "The ultimate goal of this process is to increase people's willingness to have thoughts, feelings, and other experiences they have been working hard to avoid," wrote Anthony Biglan, Steven C. Hayes, and Jacqueline Pistorello in the journal *Prevention Science*. "Efforts to control unwanted thoughts and feelings, also referred to as experiential avoidance, appear to be associated with a diverse array of psychological and behavioral difficulties," they explain. So, instead of focusing attention on trying to eliminate troublesome beliefs (the focus of CBT), ACT emphasizes learning how particular thoughts and feelings have worked (or not worked) for the individual and then encouraging the individual to commit to making conscious change.

ACT has proven to be helpful for the treatment of anxiety, depression, OCD, self-harm, substance abuse, and psychosis in children and adolescents. Typically, the language and concepts are simplified when ACT is offered to younger children (starting at age 7), while there is a greater focus, when it is offered to adolescents, on living according to your values. If applied to behavioral parent skills training, ACT can increase its impact and effectiveness.

According to Biglan, Hayes, and Pistorello, these programs tend to focus on teaching specific parenting skills, as opposed to considering parents' thoughts and feelings or their underlying values and beliefs about parenting. In society, parents are frequently encouraged to suppress negative thoughts about their children—something that encourages these thoughts to become even more intense. (As we will discuss at greater length in Chapter 5, the more you try to suppress a thought, the more intrusive it becomes.) A wiser and more effective approach, according to these authors, is to "encourage parents to accept upsetting thoughts and feelings that often accompany parenthood" while "gently challeng[ing] the assumption they must believe those thoughts or eliminate them before they can move toward parenting practices that are more effective and more in keeping with their values."

## Behavioral Activation (BA)

Proven effective for depression

BA is a treatment for depression that encourages people to change their behavior to change their thinking and their moods. It encourages them to participate in activities, even if they don't feel like it, so that they can break free of the cycle of avoidance and withdrawal that can quickly start feeding on itself when someone is depressed. The aim of the therapy is to help the individual being treated (typically a teenager, but sometimes a preteen) to make the connection between being involved in activities that they enjoy and improved mood.

## Interpersonal Psychotherapy (IPT)

Proven effective for depression

IPT is a treatment for depression that focuses on relationships with family and friends. It encourages the child (typically a preteen or teen) to consider how relationships with other people can affect her mood and behavior and how her mood and behavior can affect her relationships with other people.

## Exposure and Response Prevention (ERP)

Proven effective for OCD, social anxiety, specific phobias, panic disorder, and generalized anxiety disorder in children over age 8 and teens

ERP is a type of behavioral therapy that involves exposing the child, in a controlled setting and in a controlled manner, to things that trigger her anxiety and then preventing her from engaging in the types of rituals she has been using to manage her fears so that she can gradually learn to tolerate those feelings without the learned response. ERP can help children (age 8 and up) and teenagers who struggle with OCD, social anxiety, specific phobias, panic disorder, and generalized anxiety disorder.

## Mindfulness-Based Therapies

As the name implies, mindfulness-based therapies combine therapeutic practices with mindfulness meditation. Mindfulness-based cognitive therapy (MBCT) was designed to help people who have experienced recurrent episodes of depression, but it has been applied to other disorders as well. Mindfulness-based stress reduction (MBSR) combines mindfulness meditation and yoga. Mindfulness-based therapies are typically offered to preteens and teenagers, as opposed to younger children.

## Family Therapy

**Proven helpful for many family issues**

*Family therapy* is a generic term that is used to describe any sort of therapy that you participate in as a family (as opposed to therapy that involves your child only or that limits you to the role of support person). Family therapy gives members an opportunity to discuss and work on issues that are affecting the entire family (for example, dealing with a family member's mental illness), and the types of parenting strategies that are likely to be most effective in helping a child with mental health challenges. Family therapy is recommended in a wide variety of situations and is suitable for the families of even very young children.

Most family therapy is based on the family systems model: the belief that a family is a system and that one family member's difficulties in functioning affect all other members of the family.

That said, there are many different types of family therapy—just as there are many different types of individual therapy—with each offering its own unique focus and approach to treatment. See the appendices for more information.

> In traditional Mohawk society, anytime someone is sick, the family is healed, not just the person. That's so profound.
> **Stephanie, mother of Braeden, who has been diagnosed with OCD and ADHD**

## Group Therapy

**Proven helpful in offering peer support, communication opportunities, and normalization of mental health challenges**

Like *family therapy, group therapy* is a generic term. It refers to any sort of therapy that is offered to a group of people, as opposed to an individual. It may be led by one or more therapists and tends to have a specific focus, such as working on social skills or learning how to live well with a mental health, neurodevelopmental, or behavioral challenge. Groups are effective because they allow children to build relationships with peers who are living with the same types of challenges; encourage frank and open communication in a safe environment; and help children understand that being diagnosed with a mental health, neurodevelopmental, or behavioral challenge doesn't mean that there is something wrong with them. Groups for children and teenagers are often activity based, with therapy sometimes being offered in a camp or club setting.

### Parenting Skills Training

Proven helpful for improving family relationships

This therapeutic practice is different from family therapy, although it may be offered in conjunction with family therapy. Parenting skills training (sometimes called psychosocial training) involves teaching parents the skills they need to manage challenging types of behaviors and to strengthen family relationships. Parenting skills training is useful in a wide range of situations and is suitable for parents of even very young children.

 **NOTE:** It simply isn't possible to cover every potential treatment for every possible condition in a book of this scope. See the appendices for information about other treatment options, including links to websites where you can do some additional research.

## Hospital-Based Treatment and Residential Treatment

Depending on your child's needs, residential treatment in a mental health facility operated by trained staff or inpatient treatment on a psychiatric ward might be recommended. It's an extreme measure intended for extreme situations, but sometimes a family simply runs out of options. Mark recalls the circumstances that led to his son, Dawson, who was diagnosed with reactive attachment disorder, anxiety disorder, and moderate developmental disability, spending time in a residential treatment facility: "We realized that we needed to take a far more clinical approach. Being in a regular home environment was not conducive to treating his reactive attachment disorder. That, the onset of puberty, and ineffective medications meant that he needed something more than what we could offer at home. My husband and I are each well over six feet tall—big guys—and yet we could not stop Dawson when the rage took hold, regardless of any crisis management technique that we could employ. It was as if something took control of his body and mind—as if we weren't dealing with our son anymore." While it was difficult to consider residential treatment, the intervention made a huge difference for Mark's family: "This was a life-changer for us. Not a lot of people really understood, but not a lot of people know what reactive attachment disorder is [see Appendix A for a description] and what it does to the wiring paths of your brain. But we felt it was what he needed. It also gave us time to heal and to focus on positive interactions as a family."

## The Great Medication Debate

Depending on the nature and severity of your child's difficulties, psychiatric medications may be part of the treatment plan. Medications are often prescribed to treat the symptoms of anxiety disorders, ADHD, bipolar disorder, major depressive disorder (MDD), psychotic disorders, and schizophrenia. Medication is rarely the first option considered (unless a child's symptoms are severe). And it shouldn't be considered a stand-alone treatment. Instead, it should be combined with other treatments such as therapy (individual, group, or family), behavioral parent skills training, and educational supports. "It's a combination of medication and strategies," explains Cheyenne, whose daughter, Keisha, has been diagnosed with ADHD and anxiety. "There's not one magic pill that's going to fix it. That's what I thought in the beginning."

Before you make a decision about whether or not medication is the best option for your child, you'll want to learn as much as you can about the medication that your child's doctor is recommending. Here are some questions to ask:

- "What are the benefits of this particular medication? How likely is it to make my child's life better, and in what ways?"
- "What made you decide to recommend this particular medication as opposed to other medications that could be prescribed for this particular condition?"
- "What is the name of this medication? Are there generic versions of this medication? Do all versions of this medication work in the same way?"
- "How does the medication work?"
- "When and how does my child take this medication? What is the starting dose? How likely is that to change?"
- "Should the medication be taken with or without food?"
- "Are there any types of foods or drink that need to be avoided while my child is taking this medication? What about other medications (over-the-counter and prescription) and herbal products?"
- "If my child has difficulty swallowing pills, are there any other options?"
- "What are the known risks?"

- "What types of side effects might my child experience? What can be done to minimize those side effects?"
- "How long will it take for us to begin to notice benefits from the medication?"
- "How long will my child have to take the medication?"
- "What will you be doing to monitor the effects of this medication on my child?"
- "How often will he be seen for follow-up appointments?"
- "Who can I call if I have questions or concerns about this medication?"
- "What do I need to know about stopping this medication? Will my child have to be eased off this medication gradually?"
- "Where can I learn more about this medication?"

 **NOTE:** For help in making sense of the answers to these questions, you may want to consult *Straight Talk about Psychiatric Medications for Kids, Fourth Edition*, by Timothy E. Wilens and Paul G. Hammerness.

You will also want to ensure that you feel confident in your child's diagnosis, particularly if your child has been diagnosed with a condition requiring psychiatric medications with multiple side effects. Ellen Leibenluft, chief of the Section on Bipolar Spectrum Disorders in the Emotion and Development Branch of the National Institute of Mental Health (NIMH), urges particular caution if a child has received a diagnosis of bipolar disorder. She explains: "One thing I would say to an American parent whose child has been diagnosed with bipolar disorder is to make sure it's the right diagnosis." According to Leibenluft, "Children with severe irritability who don't have distinctive mania or hypomania are being diagnosed with bipolar disorder" and yet, clinically speaking, a bipolar diagnosis should be applied only to children who have experienced a distinct episode (either hypomania or a full-blown mania). If your child has received a bipolar diagnosis but hasn't experienced such an episode, this is something you will want to talk to your physician about: "A lot of the medications that are used to treat bipolar disorder—and that are important to use in children with bipolar disorder—have significant side effects. If the child doesn't have bipolar disorder but instead has irritability or major depression or anxiety, the medications that can be used may have fewer side effects."

**NOTE:** Some children with extreme irritability and severe tantrums meet the criteria for a brand-new diagnosis—disruptive mood dysregulation disorder (DMDD). It was added to DSM-5 to describe children who would otherwise meet the criteria for a bipolar diagnosis except for the fact that they aren't subject to manias or hypomanias.

*Speaking of Side Effects . . .*

If your child is experiencing side effects like restlessness, irritability, drowsiness, fatigue, dry mouth, trembling, memory lapses, blurred vision, and fuzzy thinking, talk to your child's doctor. It could be that such side effects will ease over time. Or it could be that your child would benefit from a change in dosage or a switch to a different medication (or a different formulation of the same medication). Your child's doctor might also recommend some specific strategies for dealing with the side effects (for example, having dinner a little later so that the medication can wear off first, if your child is struggling with a reduced appetite; administering the medication earlier in the day if your child is having trouble falling asleep; taking the medication after breakfast, if taking the medication on an empty stomach is triggering nausea, stomach pain, or headaches).

*No Easy Answers*

When you're trying to make up your mind about how to proceed, remember that you can always commit to a trial of medication for a fixed period of time to see if it makes a difference for your child and what side effects your child experiences. The length of time required varies according to the type of medication, and certain types of medications need to be phased in slowly over time. Then, with more facts in hand, you can decide whether or not the benefits outweigh the negatives and how to proceed from that point.

If you do decide to go the medication route, understand that it can take time to zero in on the right medication and the optimal dose. "It took about 18 months from diagnosis to calibrate her meds and stabilize her moods," notes Kristina about daughter Clare.

And understand that you're likely to experience mixed emotions about having to go this route. "It was terrifying every time one of his medications was taken off the market due to concerns regarding side effects, and we would become anxious and concerned and second-guess our

We initially resisted getting medication for our youngest child, not wanting to overmedicate her. But she was simply unable to regulate her emotions without the medication, which we started when she was 10. Looking back now, I realize we should have started her on medication sooner—especially since it took trying several different medications to find what worked best for her.

**Eve, mother of Tanya, Vika, and Sveta, who are dealing with adoption-related trauma and behavioral issues**

choice every time. It was a roller coaster," recalls Leigh, mother of Skyler, who has been diagnosed with ADHD, anxiety, and depression.

The good news is that sometimes medication can make a world of difference for a child and a family who are struggling. "It was like flipping a light switch rather than stumbling in the dark with matches and candles," notes Bob, whose son Steve has been diagnosed with bipolar disorder with psychotic features.

## Talking to Your Child about Treatment

It's important to talk to your child about what he can expect from treatment: what types of treatment are being planned, what they will be like, and how you hope they will make his life better.

If your child is old enough (a preteen or teenager) and developmentally capable, you may want to take things one step further by encouraging him to be actively involved in decisions about his treatment. Sometimes, out of fear that our children will make choices that we might not agree with, we are tempted to cut our children out of discussions about treatment options and to make decisions on their behalf without their explicit consent. It may be tempting to go this route, particularly if you are terrified that your child might opt out of medication or therapy that you believe he needs. But the short-term benefits that may appear to come from pressuring a child into agreeing to a particular course of treatment mean little if your child is only going through the motions. It is much healthier in terms of your child's long-term mental well-being to empower him to start making his own treatment decisions—once he is old enough and well enough, of course. Not only will you be helping him develop the skills needed to evaluate treatment options throughout his life, he'll feel more confident and in control over his life right now, at least in part because of the confidence you are demonstrating in his ability to make wise choices. The alternative—coercing your child into agreeing to treatment options that he doesn't believe are right for him—can be damaging to his self-esteem and to your relationship with one another.

That said, when you're dealing with a younger child (as opposed to a preteen or teenager), you may have to emphasize the benefits of treatment when making the case for various treatment options.

Christine remembers the conversations she had with her son, Will—who was then 7—about the therapy and medication that were part of his treatment plan for severe ADHD and an anxiety disorder: "I told Will that his therapist was simply someone he could talk to. I told him he could tell his therapist anything and it would always be private. I made sure he knew that the therapist couldn't share anything with me or with his school unless he gave his permission. Will loved the idea of having someone he could talk to about anything, and who wouldn't share any of his secrets, so that went well."

Their conversation about medication proved to be a little more difficult. "Will couldn't understand why he had to take medication every day when none of his friends had to. He didn't feel that he was 'sick,' so why did he need medication?"

Christine ended up having to build in artificial incentives to encourage Will to take his medication until Will could start to experience the genuine incentive of feeling more in control of his life. She explains: "For the first couple of weeks, we bribed him with special treats: his favorite foods, movies, video games, anything that motivated him to take his medication that morning. After that, Will could see how much easier school was for him. He was no longer getting into trouble every day, the work was easier, he was getting along better with his friends, and he was happier. Since then, he has taken his medication willingly. I'm sure he'd rather not have to take it, but now he sees the difference it makes."

Marie recalls the medication conversation that she had with her son David, who has been diagnosed with the severe combined form of ADHD, sensory integration disorder, and two emerging learning disabilities, as "no big deal." She explains: "David has a friend who uses hearing aids, so he equated his medication to an aid, just like the hearing aid that helps his friend hear."

While Leigh's 7-year-old son, Skyler, was initially willing to take medication for his ADHD, anxiety, and depression, he changed his mind once he started to experience nasty side effects. "All the medications had side effects that were unpleasant," Leigh recalls. "Nausea, metallic taste, loss of appetite, buzzing in his head.

"This made Skyler very frustrated and angry. Taking his medication was often a battle. When he got old enough that he was hiding his medication rather than taking it, we allowed him to decide to stop taking his medication. He had become resentful of us for 'making him take meds' and, to this day, he won't even take over-the-counter medications for allergies or the occasional headache. And I became resentful that I had spent years medicating my son so that he would be more manageable in school, yet [the school] still didn't have good strategies in place, and we were somewhat back where we started but with an older, more frustrated young man."

When you're dealing with an older child or adolescent, it's important to involve him in treatment decisions as much as possible, says Andrew, whose son David has been diagnosed with schizophrenia. "Be direct and hopeful with your child when presenting treatment options. Be encouraging and supportive throughout. The more responsibility they can take for their treatment, the better—but most children with serious mental health problems will need ongoing help."

"Offer and encourage treatment, but don't make it a battle," advises Michelle, who has one son diagnosed with depression with suicidal thoughts and another son diagnosed with generalized anxiety disorder. "This will only make things worse." And, ultimately, if things do turn into a battle, you'll quickly discover that it's a battle you simply can't win. Eve explains: "All three of my children with mental health issues dramatically resisted treatment. None of them would talk to a therapist. None of them wanted to take medication and would lie, saying they'd taken it when they hadn't. Seeking treatment for my children brought out extremely oppositional behavior in them all, and it was exhausting and demoralizing for me, and (12 years into this experience) remains so. It felt like money wasted, and yet not trying anything wasn't an option, given their behavior at home, at school, and in the world."

Understanding that children and adolescents think differently than adults may help you feel at least a little less frustrated by the situation. In other words, don't expect a young teenager to be able to judiciously weigh the pros and cons of a decision like medication use in quite the same way you can. "Young teenagers will mainly believe what they can see or have experienced and, thus, they cannot fully appreciate the long-term or unseen consequences of not taking their medications," wrote Danielle Taddeo, Maud Egedy, and Jean-Yves Frappier in an article published in *Paediatrics and Child Health*. It's important to respect the fact that while clinicians may be experts when it comes to the disease and its treatment, "the teen is the expert of his or her own life and priorities," they note. If your child's therapist and doctor—and you, her parent—are able to respond to her resistance to taking medication with "a nonjudgmental approach characterized by warmth, respect, and empathy, but also curiosity (interest in the adolescent's view), low investment (which involves . . . exploring, accepting, and trying to understand the adolescent's view rather than coercing them to change attitudes and behaviors) and flexibility," you may be able to find some workable solutions together.

Children and teenagers are more likely to agree to take their medication if they feel that their concerns about medication use are being taken seriously. Here's what this means in practical terms:

- You acknowledge that the side effects can be annoying.
- You remind your child that the advantages of taking the medication appear to outweigh the disadvantages.
- You promise to review the issue of medication use with her doctor at her next appointment.

It is important to have this kind of conversation with your child as opposed to simply ordering her to take the medication. You want to encourage your child to be an active participant in her own health care decisions as opposed to simply passively going along with any health recommendations that are offered to her. And, ultimately, your child can find a way to do an end run around you on the medication front, should she choose to do so (by hiding the medication under her tongue, in her cheek, in her bedroom closet, and so forth, while cheerfully reassuring you that she swallowed it).

> With schizophrenia, part of the disease is often an inability to recognize that you are ill or to admit that there is a problem. My son took his meds while denying he had schizophrenia. When asked why, he said that the meds made him feel better.
> **Marvin, father of David**

Many parents find that therapy alone is sufficient to treat their child's disorder. Others find that, once they've made the tough decision to add medication to the treatment mix, things begin to get a lot better for their children and their families.

"The diagnosis has improved my son's quality of life to no bounds," says Mara, whose son, Jake, has been diagnosed with ADHD. "The medication allows him to function in 'polite society.' With his impulse control problems (combined with his giftedness), he was having major social issues. Kids just didn't want to be around him. He was irritating, loud, and would sometimes hurt kids without realizing it. Now, he's just one of the guys."

"Right away, Tom felt different," recalls Kim. "His exact words were 'It's like my emotions aren't having a party in my head anymore.' That was pretty deep for a 9-year-old. Medication, combined with an understanding of ADHD by Tom and those around him, helped him to feel more confident and happier with himself."

> Antidepressants helped a lot initially. As my daughter said at the time, "Taking them makes me realize it isn't normal to have the same thought a thousand times."
> **Lily, mother of Asia, who has been diagnosed with BPD**

Marie has witnessed a similar transformation in her son. "The diagnosis and treatment led to David being able to concentrate in class, have more control over his sensory issues and needs, and, best of all, he was no longer a prisoner of his own imagination. He could no longer be dragged into his own mind against his will. He was in control. This was enormously freeing to him."

The most challenging thing about the medication issue is, for many parents, the unhelpful comments and reactions of other people. "One friend who was studying to be a naturopath has made several comments to me about a teacher of hers who says she can get anyone with ADHD off their meds with natural treatments," says Tami, whose son Adam is taking medication for ADHD. "It was not an easy decision to put Adam on medication, and these comments were not supportive in the least, although I'm sure she felt she was being helpful."

Mara doesn't have a lot of patience for such comments: "If my kid had epilepsy, I wouldn't fight a diagnosis and medication. Why should mental health be any different?"

If you find yourself dealing with unhelpful comments from family members and friends about your handling of the medication decision (you're likely to receive criticism whether you opt for medication or not, by the way), you may want to come up with some rote responses that you can rely on over and over again. "Thanks for your concern, but we have spent a lot of time researching this issue, and we feel that we've made the decision that's right for our family and our child" is the type of response that works well for many families. You are giving the advice giver the benefit of the doubt when it comes to his or her intentions—you're assuming the person is acting out of genuine concern—and yet you are still standing firm with regard to your decision.

## What to Do If You're Worried about the Effectiveness of Treatment

It's been a few months—or maybe more than a few months—and you're not seeing the kind of progress you had hoped to see by now. What should you do?

### Set Up a Time to Meet with Members of Your Child's Treatment Team

You can take that opportunity to find out whether your child is progressing as well as anticipated. Perhaps your child's therapist and/or doctor shares your concerns. Ask what other treatment options they might recommend. If you are the parent of an older teen or young adult, you will have to ask your child to give his treatment team permission to involve you in treatment discussions (the downside of health privacy legislation) or to share information about his progress with you. But don't let that stop you from sharing any relevant information with them. There's no law stating you can't share information (perhaps via a letter) with your child's doctor; privacy legislation simply prevents them from communicating about your child with you. (See Chapters 4 and 14 for more about this issue.)

### *Realize That This Is a Common— Albeit Frustrating—Experience*

Human beings aren't nearly as predictable as machines. Input doesn't always predict output. Sometimes a whole lot of tweaking is required before treatment begins to produce the desired solutions. And sometimes, even with that tweaking, you're still left far short of the goal.

"We have found the various treatments available so far to be unpredictable as to what might work or not," says Andrew. "Often what seems like reasonable treatment is limited by various factors and one has to settle for something less than hoped for. Side effects are often a concern and one must do a cost–benefit analysis as to whether to take a certain course of action. Some treatments may appear to work for a while but then appear to stop helping. This can be discouraging."

You may also be frustrated to discover that a treatment recognized as the gold standard of treatment for your child's condition simply doesn't work well for your child. There's no such thing as a one-size-fits-all treatment solution—and there certainly isn't anything even remotely resembling a one-type-works-for-all magic little pill.

You may be shocked (and a bit overwhelmed) to discover just how vital you are to the success of the treatment process. "The most surprising aspect of this journey has been learning that, in the end, we are the ones who have had to figure out what works best for our children," says Susan, whose son Jacob struggles with anxiety. "I think we thought that the professionals would tell us what was wrong and how to fix it. Ultimately, we decided what worked best for our son and then enlightened the professionals."

Priya, whose son Ravi has been diagnosed with Asperger syndrome, had a similar experience. Don't wait for someone else to step in and save your kid, she urges other parents. Be prepared to do that heavy lifting yourself: "We were still in this mode of believing, '*Somebody* knows better what to do than we do. *Somebody* will save us.' Then finally one day we realized that you have to be prepared to save your kid yourself."

## What to Do If You're Worried about the Quality of Treatment

There's no denying it: sometimes the mental health care system lets families down. And when it does, it tends to do so in a big way.

---

### Privacy and Adolescents

Privacy concerns may prevent clinicians from providing you with detailed information about your adolescent or young adult, but that doesn't prevent you from passing along information that you think they need to know to assess and treat your child. For example, you can provide updates on how your child is functioning at home, at school, and in the community. You can also continue to encourage your teenager or young adult to involve you in the treatment process by showing him how much you care and how eager you are to support his recovery.

---

That has certainly been Marvin's experience. He describes himself as a "mental health street fighter" as a result of the battles he's been forced to fight on behalf of his son David. He explains, "Medication is the foundation for treatment of schizophrenia, and when David was first referred to a case management program, they were very good at getting him back to school and referring him to a job program for people with disabilities. Meaningful activity over and above just giving meds is essential. We've noticed that this emphasis is now gone. That has led to many fights with the system. . . . It is a constant fight where I am told they cannot talk to me because my son is over 18. All of this is very time-consuming and stressful, but if it is not done, then nothing is done for my son."

Lydia, whose son Thomas has struggled with suicidal feelings, can certainly relate to Marvin's sense of frustration. "Thomas went to live in a group home from the age of 14 to the age of 17. While he was there, he bonded with a counselor who took the time to really understand him and get him the supports he needed with regard to counseling and education. Once he left that facility, all his supports were gone and there was no referral made for continued counseling. He ended up in jail for 3 months because he was self-medicating with street drugs. This had a huge impact on our family and was one of the issues that really tore us apart."

The type of fallout that Lydia's family experienced when her son transitioned from one type of care to another is, unfortunately, not uncommon. If you have the luxury of knowing ahead of time that your child will be moving from one type of care to another (for example, your child will be moving from the child and youth mental health system to the adult mental health system because of his age), you can sometimes help to ease the transition by initiating the search for new services far ahead of time. It is a good idea to start inquiring about mental health services for your soon-to-be young adult (*emerging adult* is the term that gets used a lot these days) when he or she turns seventeen. That way, you'll have an entire year to find appropriate adult programs and supports to replace the existing programs and supports that your child is going to have to leave behind. (See Chapter 13 for more about helping your child to thrive during the transition to young adulthood.)

Sadly, many parents who have been through negative experiences with the mental health system have come away with the feeling of being blamed unfairly for any failures in the process. "I learned that a lot of professionals think parents are idiots," confirms Tara, whose son Aiden has been diagnosed with autism and ODD and whose son Owen has been diagnosed with anxiety and ADHD. "Other parents need to know that they shouldn't take that personally. It isn't just them. Fortunately, there are a lot of really great people working in the system. You just have to find them."

Like Tara, Andrew believes that it's important to hang tough despite a bad experience. Not only is your child counting on you to find the right help, *there is help available.* "It may take time to access what you need. Don't give up, and don't paint the whole system with a negative brush if you have some frustrating experiences or meet some unhelpful professionals along the way. Stay positive and keep an open mind. . . . Try to stay grateful for the good things that are available to you, because no matter how bad you might think the system is now, it's a lot better than it was just a few decades ago."

> You'll make a lot of phone calls and wait for a lot of callbacks that don't come half the time. Write down a script ahead of time. Recognize that this is emotionally hard for you, too. To the receptionist you're just making an appointment. But you're scared and worried and alone and no one gives a f———. You need to let yourself have a good cry or dinner with a friend or whatever.
>
> **Jennifer, mother of Jessica**

## How to Get Support

It's easy to become so focused on trying to meet your child's needs that you overlook your own need for support during this challenging time. It is important to remind yourself that taking good care of yourself is one of the most important things you can do to help your child.

### Reach Out

To help yourself stay strong while you're advocating for your child, try reaching out for support from other parents who are walking the same walk. Organizations such as the National Alliance on Mental Illness (*www. nami.org*) and the Federation of Families for Children's Mental Health (*www. ffcmh.org*) can help you to make connections. See Appendix B at the back of the book for additional organizations that offer or can refer you to sources of support. Other families can share insider advice on making the system work for you. Don't be afraid to speak up (in a respectful and solutions-oriented manner) about what's not working for your family with your child's mental health treatment. If that doesn't resolve the problem to your satisfaction, find out to whom the clinician reports and take your issues up with that person. Repeat this process until your concerns have been addressed and your child is receiving the high-caliber treatment he deserves.

### Look into Counseling for You

You might find it helpful to go for individual or couple counseling to deal with feelings about your child's diagnosis or to sort out parenting conflicts that have arisen while you and your partner have been trying to deal with your child's behavior. David's father, Andrew, found it helpful to participate in both types of therapy. "Family therapy can be a useful thing. Parents can go for their own therapy to try to figure out how to best help their child and manage their unfolding grief and anxiety. This can be done with an individual therapist, but there are also parent support groups for this kind of situation, which can be helpful. The whole family system needs adequate support along with the child in treatment," he explains.

Tapping into that type of support—and dealing with your thoughts and feelings head-on—will lead to a stronger, healthier you. And that is great news for your child and your family. "You are the glue that holds your family together," explains Grace, whose oldest son, Alex, has been diagnosed with Asperger syndrome. "You have to do whatever you can to keep that glue strong."

See Chapter 4 for more advice on tapping into support and becoming the best possible advocate for your child.

# 4

# Advocating for Your Child

From the time your parent radar alerts you to the fact that your child is struggling, you become your child's advocate within the health care system and, for school-age children, the school system as well. That means taking a leadership role in gathering information and keeping records, asking insistently for the help you know your child needs (and taking into account what she tells you she

> You need to push. You need to be the squeaky wheel. You need to demand the best for your child. Adequate is not good enough.
> **Marie, mother of David, who has been diagnosed with the severe combined form of ADHD, sensory integration disorder, and two learning disabilities**

needs), continuing to ask questions until you get satisfactory answers, and generally doing everything you can to help your child as she makes her way through these complex and often confusing systems. Your child needs a strong advocate—someone who can represent her interests and act as her voice when decisions need to be made. Because you know your child best, you're the best person to take on that role until she's old enough and well enough to take it on for herself.

And you do want her to take on this role for herself, as soon as she is able, so that she can begin to develop the skills needed to speak out about what she needs from you, her teachers, the members of her mental health care team, your insurance provider, and other significant people in her life.

The best way to encourage her to develop these skills is by giving her the chance to work on them with you at home, so that she feels safe and supported about speaking up about what she wants and needs. For this type of dialogue to occur, she needs to know that you will:

- Listen, without judgment, to what she has to say.
- Treat her thoughts and ideas with respect (both her worries and concerns and her hopes and dreams for herself).
- Provide her with constructive and encouraging feedback as she works at developing her self-advocacy skills.

If you're a naturally assertive person, taking on the role of advocate will feel comfortable to you right away—like stepping into a second skin. If you're a little more reserved, it may take you a bit of time to grow into the role—but know that you have what it takes. "Don't be afraid to advocate for your children in every system that they touch," says Darcy Gruttadaro, director of NAMI's Child and Adolescent Action Center in Arlington, Virginia. "You have to be your child's best advocate."

Unsure how to get started? Worried that you're not up to the task? Here are a few tips.

## Advocacy 101

### Recognize That This Is Hard Work

Advocating for your child can be physically and emotionally draining. To do the best possible job of advocating for your child, you need to do an even better job of caring for yourself. That means treating self-care as a necessity, not a luxury. After all, no one needs a healthy parent more than a child who is struggling. (See Chapters 1, 5, and 9 and the section at the end of this chapter for more on this all-important topic.)

It's also important to recognize that you don't have to do this on your own. Connect with other parents who have figured out how the educational and health care systems work in your part of the world—and who can shorten your learning curve. If it takes a village to raise a child, it takes a village to support that parent. Don't be afraid to turn to your village for support as you do the hard work of advocating for your child. (See Chapter 12 for more about tapping into support.)

### Trust Your Gut

A parent's intuition is a powerful force. Trust it to tell you when you need to speak up on your child's behalf. "Be the mama bear. If something isn't right in your gut, it isn't right," says Michelle, whose son John has been diagnosed with depression with suicidal thoughts and whose son Martin has been diagnosed with generalized anxiety disorder. "The teacher has a whole different class next year. The doctor has 500 patients. Your child only has you."

## Learn How the Systems Work

The best way to help your child obtain the best possible mental health care and the best possible support at school is to understand how the mental health and school systems work in the part of the country where you live. Visit national, state, and county websites to learn how the systems are structured and what services are available to your child. ("Services can even vary on a county-to-county basis," notes Ruby, mother of two children with autism spectrum disorders and other challenges.) And spend time exploring mental health association websites and parent advocacy group websites to find out what other supports are available to your child and your family, both in person and online. "Know that you're not alone," says Gruttadaro. "Connect with people who have walked in your shoes—who have great advice and great ideas and also who are active in advocacy because they want a better mental health system for all children." Note: You'll find additional tips on navigating the school system in Chapter 10 plus a detailed discussion of what it will take to create a more family-friendly mental health care system in Chapter 14.

## Tap into the Expertise of Other People

Ask lots of questions at your child's school and of your child's treatment team—and don't be afraid to seek assistance from anyone else who might be able to help you tap into the right services and supports. "For complicated types of situations, the child psychiatry departments of university medical schools are good places to start," says Ellen Leibenluft, chief of the Section on Bipolar Spectrum Disorders at the Emotion and Development Branch of the NIMH.

If you are feeling intimidated by the process, consider taking a support person with you to important meetings—someone who is familiar with the process and who can help you function at your best. You can ask that person to take detailed notes during the meeting so you can focus on establishing relationships with the other people around the table and making the best possible case for your child. And don't be afraid to seek the services of an educational consultant or other person with experience helping families navigate the school and mental health systems. "Having an informed third-party adviser was critical when Jess was younger," says Jennifer, whose daughter, Jessica, experiences a variety of physical and mental health difficulties related to tuberous sclerosis. "I met an amazing speech therapist when Jess was about 3, through an early childhood intervention program the school district provided. When Jess outgrew that program, the speech therapist was still my adviser. She was accustomed to dealing with IEP meetings and schools, and whenever I had a problem she was able to offer advice. She also had a good sense of what battles were worth fighting."

### Do Your Homework

Learn as much as you can about the specific challenges your child is dealing with. That way you can hold your own during discussions with your child's school and mental health care team. Keep a running list of questions in a notebook and keep asking those questions until you're satisfied with the answers you've received.

### Stay on Top of the Process

Know what is supposed to be happening next for your child—and by what date—and follow up with service providers to ensure that your child's treatment stays on track. "Respectfully fight for follow-up," says Stephanie, whose son Braeden has been diagnosed with OCD and ADHD. "Make sure referrals are sent in a timely manner. Push (nicely) for your child to be seen."

### Maintain Meticulous Records

Don't rely on your child's doctor, your child's school, or anyone else to keep track of your child's mental health history. Keep your own detailed set of records (see the section on record keeping later in this chapter). Someone working with your child might ask for specific details about your child's medical or educational history, and that information is easier to provide if you have it at your fingertips. You need to have your own set of accurate records to advocate effectively on behalf of your child. "Buy a notebook and a binder and document every meeting and phone conversation," says Laura, whose son, Gabriel, has been diagnosed with Asperger syndrome (a diagnosis that has been changed to autism spectrum disorder in DSM-5) and is currently being assessed for OCD. "Do research and keep documents in the binder. Follow up on things and ask lots of questions. If your child had cancer, you would stop at nothing to get them the treatment needed. The same should be true of mental health. It's a health care issue, plain and simple."

Rebecca, whose daughter, Madalyn, has been diagnosed with learning disabilities and is currently awaiting a follow-up assessment to better pinpoint the full scope of her difficulties, has taken this approach as well. "I've become this machine," she says. "I scan and save all the documents I receive or forms I fill out and put them on Google Drive so I can easily access them and share them. And I recently started a spreadsheet tracking all the calls I make so I can make sure I don't drop the ball."

## Be Prepared

Spend some time thinking about what you want for your child before you head into important meetings. You'll be a more effective advocate if you have a specific goal in mind (you know what your child needs and you have thoughts about how that need might be met) and you have a list of questions to ask and concerns to discuss. This helps both to keep the meeting on track and to keep yourself from reacting emotionally in the moment in a way that might not be helpful to your child or family. It also helps to boost your credibility and your confidence: "The more you can learn first and be a well-educated consumer, the better, because then you go in with a voice of authority," says Gruttadaro.

## Remind Yourself That How You Communicate Is As Important As What You Say

Try to remain positive and focus on finding solutions rather than assigning blame, no matter how frustrated you may be with the school or mental health system. "A voice of authority, leading with respect for those you are working with, will go a long way toward getting what your child needs," notes Gruttadaro.

## Involve Your Child As Much As Possible

If he is not yet old enough to advocate for himself, involve him in decision making in an age-appropriate way. "Self-advocacy, being able to speak on your own behalf, is an important life skill," note Helen Parker, Janet Phillips, and Cathy Bedard in *Speaking Up! A Parent Guide to Advocating for Students in Public Schools*. "For students to be effective as self-advocates, parents and all other adults need to accept a child's right to be treated with respect and dignity. Adults also need to accept that children have the right to have their views carefully considered when decisions are made about them." If your child is still too young to attend meetings on his own behalf, ask for his input in advance so you can be his voice at the meeting. If that is not possible, try to see the world through his eyes and think about what he would want you to say. Look for opportunities to allow his voice to be present at the table, even if he can't be there in person. Help him write a letter or draw a picture expressing his concerns, if he is able, or take notes on his behalf while he is talking about what he wants and needs. You might even consider inviting him to speak to the other people around the table via a short video that you can play at the meeting. It's a powerful way to give him a voice and to give other people who haven't had the privilege of meeting him a fuller sense of who he is as a person.

### Know When It's Time to Bump Things Up a Level

"Don't be afraid to move up the ladder if you're not getting what you need," says Gruttadaro. "Use all the resources available to you." Sure, you want to respect protocols (because escalating your concerns to the next level prematurely is more likely to work against your family than for it). But it's also important to know when it's time to get other people—including politicians—involved, she explains. "I tell families, 'Contact your state representative. Contact your county government. Contact your federal legislator. They are there to represent you. That's why we call them representatives.'"

Of course, timing is everything when it comes to advocacy. You don't want to be overly aggressive by jumping up a level until you've exhausted all opportunities to make progress with the people you are working with. But once you've done that, and you haven't gotten what your child needs, don't be afraid to write a letter to the people you've been working with, documenting your experiences and highlighting the areas where your child's needs have not been met—and then copying the right people (people who can make a difference for your child) on that letter. "Be very savvy and be very smart about how you do this," Gruttadaro cautions, noting that families are understandably afraid to speak up in case someone decides to retaliate against their child. "They say things like 'I don't want them to dig in and further deny our family care.'" If you're not quite sure how to proceed, think about reaching out to NAMI, particularly at the affiliate and state levels, for help in advocating for your child. "They understand what's available and what's possible at the state and local levels. They know the clinicians and the system—and they know how to work it—and they can help guide you through this process. You don't have to go this alone."

# Record Keeping for Advocacy Purposes

You will find it easier to advocate for your child if you make a point of maintaining detailed records for your child on an ongoing basis. You may find it works well to create a binder for this purpose and to divide the binder into the following categories, so that you can organize existing information and add to this record over time. You can also use the downloadable forms available at *www.guilford.com/douglas-forms* (print, complete, and keep them in your binder or fill them out and keep them up to date and stored electronically).

## Contacts

Keep the contact information (phone number, email, agency, and mailing address) for the mental health professionals involved in diagnosing and treating your child. Include the names and job titles of key contacts at your child's school (classroom teacher, special education teacher, principal).

## Medical and Developmental History

This is where details about your child's medical and developmental history go, including a copy of your child's birth certificate and important details related to pregnancy, birth, and early development. Include details about childhood illnesses, medical assessments, diagnoses, and treatments.

## Educational History

Keep details about your child's school history here, including report cards, records of educational assessments and standardized tests, correspondence with the school, and incident reports. If your child has been suspended from school or experienced other significant incidents, describe the incident that occurred, using your child's own words, and note how the incident was handled by the school and any disciplinary action that was taken.

## Symptom Notes

Record the date of the onset of symptoms (or a change in the nature of symptoms) and make notes about the severity of symptoms and about any possible triggers.

## Treatment Notes

Include notes about the different approaches to treatment that have been tried. Record the dates that the treatment started and ended, the name of the treatment provider (the doctor and agency), a brief description of the nature of the treatment (type of therapy, medication type and dosage), and a description of the outcome (was this treatment successful?).

### Meeting and Phone Call Notes

Include notes you made during meetings at school, meetings with your child's doctor, meetings with mental health care providers, and any phone calls related to your child's education or mental health treatment. Be sure to record the date of all meetings and any decisions made or actions resulting from such meetings, so that you can remember to follow up later on.

### Research Notes

Include information about your child's diagnoses, details about your child's treatment, and parenting information that you find useful.

### Individualized Education Program

Keep a copy of your child's IEP on file.

### Crisis Plan

In this section, write down your child's triggers (events, experiences, and emotions that have led to symptoms in the past) and effective strategies for coping with triggers. Record the early warning signs (specific to your child) that she may be experiencing a worsening of symptoms—and how to respond.

### Recovery Plan

Make notes about your child's strengths and abilities, coping strategies, hopes and dreams, short-term and long-term goals, and any other information that could be used to help your child identify and set recovery goals (see Chapter 13).

## Feeling Let Down by the System

Advocating for your child is hard work. It can be time-consuming and frustrating. And it can leave you feeling let down by a system (or nonsystem) that isn't working nearly well enough to meet the needs of children and their parents. But it certainly beats the alternative—feeling completely defeated by the situation. "I had been feeling very helpless before I became an advocate," explains Liza Long, author of *The Price of Silence,* and mother of a teenager who has been diagnosed with bipolar disorder. "Advocacy is doing something. Maybe you can't change the world, but at least you're trying and at least you're doing something instead of just sitting there and saying, 'This is hopeless.'"

Of course, there are days when the situation can feel pretty hopeless. According to the Bazelon Center for Mental Health Law, "Mental disorders affect about one in five American children, yet only about a fifth of these children actually receive the mental health services they need." And here's the ugly truth hidden in that statistic: lengthy waits to access treatment cause real harm to children, contributing to clinical deterioration and an increased risk of suicide or hospitalization.

It can be shocking to discover that your child is faced with a lengthy wait for service when she is dealing with a pressing mental health problem right now. "Children need access to help immediately, not in 6 months," says Sari, mother of Ryan, who has been diagnosed with ADHD, and Emma, who has been diagnosed with ADHD and anxiety.

The issue of children receiving only partial treatment as opposed to the kind of treatment they actually need must also be addressed, she adds: "Children need to have access to doctors and therapists on a regular basis, not once every 2 months, if that. Parents need to be able to get the support and information they need in a more organized and efficient way. Bottom line? We need more doctors, more therapists, and better organization of services."

At the heart of the problem is the fact that there's a critical shortage of child psychiatrists and other pediatric mental health professionals. "There are only 8,000 child psychiatrists in America—but between 20,000 and 30,000 are needed to meet the needs of children requiring psychiatric care," notes Gruttadaro. "Some communities are extremely underserviced. There may not even be a pediatrician in practice."

And even if there is a pediatrician or child psychiatrist practicing in your community, obtaining access to that person isn't necessarily a given. "The most infuriating part is how bureaucratic and complicated some things can be," says Laura. "We've had a fair bit of experience dealing with the mental health services where we live now and have experienced frustrations like people not calling you back, very limited hours for certain services, and so on."

And, of course, battles with insurance companies over what is and isn't covered can be legendary—even in an era of (supposed) mental health parity. Insurance companies continue to find ways to limit the costs associated with mental health treatment by limiting access to care. Common strategies include limiting the number of appointments and/or the types of medications that are covered, denying care on the grounds that it isn't medically necessary (with the insurance company making that judgment), insisting that doctor's visits for mental health reasons be preauthorized by the insurance company, and/or implementing "fail first" policies that force people to try less expensive treatments as opposed to immediately zeroing in on the optimal form of care. The strategies seem to be working—for insurance companies rather than families, that is: a 2015 study conducted by NAMI found that survey respondents were twice as likely to report being denied payment for services that were deemed "not medically necessary" when those services involved mental health services as opposed to other types of medical services.

These are battles that Jennifer has fought repeatedly on her daughter, Jessica's, behalf. Her advice? Choose your insurance company with care and understand how to make your plan work for, not against, you: "It all starts with having the right insurance company. Some are notorious for routinely denying claims they should pay because a certain percentage of people won't fight the decision. Avoid those insurance companies (easier said than done, but Google is your friend) and understand your plan—how authorizations are obtained, how much is covered, and so on. Assume the insurance company is looking for a reason to deny your claim, so make that as hard as possible for it. You may find that if services are called one thing they're covered but if they're called something else they're not. Enlist the help of your health care providers. They can often point you to low-cost alternatives and programs."

One medication that helped our daughter tremendously cost hundreds of dollars per month. We got a free trial for a year, but after that the drug company wouldn't extend it. We couldn't afford the medication, which wasn't covered by our insurance, so we had to switch to another drug, which also worked but isn't available in a one-dose-per-day pill. There is no generic form of the once-a-day pill that worked for her, because of the drug company's patent. I don't know the solution, but it seems that either insurance should cover such expensive medications for families or the drug companies should not be allowed to charge so much for them. Now my daughter takes the similar drug three times a day, but it's hard enough to get her to take pills once a day, and she often skips doses, so her impulsivity kicks in and she makes poor choices that hurt her life.

**Eve, mother of three daughters who have all experienced adoption-related trauma and behavioral issues**

There's a lot you can accomplish by being a savvy and persistent advocate—but don't expect to work miracles on the insurance front, says Jennifer: "You have to accept the reality that, in this country, mental health services are not well covered. We have good insurance, but I would actually have some retirement savings if not for Jessica's massive medical problems."

## Finding Other Allies in the Quest for Better Care

Parents aren't the only ones who are frustrated with the state of the children's mental health care system in America. You may find it comforting to know that people working in the field of child and youth mental health care are also frustrated by the current inadequacies of the system. They object to the fact that kids have to wait so long to be assessed and to access treatment. They struggle with the fact that there are fewer and fewer child psychiatrists. And they resent the fact that the system is complicated, uncoordinated, and poorly funded. They have to work around these realities every day. When it comes to dreaming of a better mental health care system for children and adolescents, we're all on the same team. See Chapter 14 for more thoughts on creating a mental health care system that truly works for children, youth, and families.

## Staying Strong

It takes energy and stamina to be able to advocate on your child's behalf over the long term. At times you may feel like you've signed up for a marathon—an emotional marathon—that is challenging you to the max. The best way to deal with that challenge is by tackling it head on—zeroing in on what you need to stay strong. That means tapping into support from family and friends, including other parents who have walked this walk, and taking the best possible care of yourself (eating well, exercising regularly, making time for fun, managing stress, and getting adequate sleep). Advocacy takes energy. Make sure you're giving yourself the physical and emotional fuel you need so you can be the strongest possible advocate for your child. See Chapters 5 and 9 for practical advice on managing stress and improving wellness.

# Part II

# You and Your Child

There might be times when you will feel utterly useless—like nothing you do or say is doing your child any good at all. Maybe you've had this humbling experience already. If so, you know exactly what I'm talking about. During times like this, it is important to remind yourself that you are making a world of difference for your child simply by offering your love and support.

This is important to keep in mind if you've been feeling discouraged or more than a little hopeless. And it's especially crucial to know if you find you've been waiting for the mental health fairy godmother to show up on your porch, wave her magic wand, and make all your family's worries disappear.

Speaking of which, I guess it's time I told you the truth about the mental health fairy godmother.

*There is no mental health fairy godmother.*

A police officer broke the news to me one night after he had helped my husband locate my daughter in the middle of the night. He was offering me his best advice on what we could do to cope with our daughter's illness: "You can't wait for someone else to step in to save your daughter. You have to save your daughter yourself."

What he said was both terrifying and liberating. Instead of waiting for some miracle solution to come to us from somewhere else— from some mental health fairy godmother—it was time to take the power back into our own hands, to realize that we could start solving this problem ourselves. After all, no one else knew our daughter as well as we did, and no one else loved her even a fraction as much. That's not to say that we walked away from the caring professionals who were working so hard to help our daughter and family. We simply stopped expecting them to be able to deliver miracle solutions overnight.

In the end, it was our daughter who saved herself (she had to want to recover to begin to make changes to her life), but we were able to provide her with the supports she needed as she readied herself to make that change. She needed to know that we were there, ready to catch her as she took those first baby steps toward a happier, healthier life.

So, what can you do to begin to make life better for yourself and your child? Plenty, as it turns out.

In addition to continuing to seek support for your child and your family, you can choose parenting strategies that will encourage your child to love and accept himself. You can work on your own stress management and coping skills and model these skills for your child. You can be present for your child and help him learn how to manage his emotions more effectively. Children at all ages are learning how to manage their feelings without squashing them or hiding them. We can model adult behavior to show them how, with compassion and understanding. These are the issues we'll be talking about in the next three chapters. And, of course, you will read about the experiences of parents who have been where you are now and hear their words of advice.

I hope I can help you avoid spiraling downward to the same extent that I did when my children were struggling. As a result of the layers upon layers of accumulated stress (plus job-related pressures and my mother's sudden and unexpected death), I ended up nosediving into a 3-year-long depression and gaining 100 pounds, which I then had to work hard to lose. So if I seem to preach self-care a little too enthusiastically in this part of the book, it's for good reason. I'm a pretty passionate convert.

# 5

# Stress Management and Coping Skills

Our brains don't function at their best when we're feeling stressed. Our thinking gets muddled and we get bogged down by negative emotion. That makes it difficult for us to take care of ourselves, let alone anyone else.

"Stress leads to a destructive cycle in the brain: depression and anxiety induce brain cell loss, which results in disturbances in thinking, concentration, memory, sleep, and general well-being. Taken together, these disturbances cycle back to produce even more stress," notes Richard Restak in his book *Think Smart: A Neuroscientist's Prescription for Improving Your Brain's Performance.*

Fortunately, there are a number of things we can do to disrupt this truly vicious cycle—a cycle that can affect us as well as our children. We can learn strategies for coping with stress. We can make a conscious effort to increase the amount of positive emotion we are experiencing. We can practice relaxation techniques that are known to help our bodies manage stress. And we can teach

> For Charlotte, it's been helpful to teach her several different forms of relaxation. It can take a while to hit on the one that works best for an individual child. It's important to have many tools in the tool box.
>
> **Alison, mother of Charlotte, who struggles with anxiety**

these techniques to our children. It's worth noting that a study published in 2012 found that children who believe that they are capable of coping with the demands of stressful situations experience fewer mental health problems than other children.

In this chapter the focus will be on helping you deal with the stress in your life without letting it overwhelm you. Remember, if you can't function effectively yourself, you can't be the caring parent and forceful advocate that you want to be and that your child needs you to be. The following suggestions for coping with stress might be useful not only to you but also to your child who is struggling and the rest of the family. Do them—and yourself—a favor by sharing these techniques.

## Shifting Your Thinking

Stress is a fact of life for those of us who have children dealing with mental health, neurodevelopmental, and behavioral challenges. While we may not be able to eliminate the source of our stress—the fact that our children are struggling—we can control the way we react to that situation. In fact, sometimes that's the only thing we can control.

Here are some strategies that other parents have found helpful.

### Learn to Recognize the Early Warning Signs That You Are Becoming Stressed

You want to avoid becoming flooded with emotion (making it impossible to react calmly and rationally) or experiencing burnout (the result of chronic, unrelenting stress). According to Stuart Shanker, author of *Calm, Alert, and Learning: Classroom Strategies for Self-Regulation,* the early warning cues are unique to each individual but may include behavioral changes (difficulty sleeping, increased or decreased appetite) as well as bodily sensations (tightness in the chest, headaches, stomachaches, and tingling in the hands and fingers). When you recognize that your stress is escalating, you can try an appropriate coping strategy. You will likely need to experiment with different techniques and activities (relaxation breathing, mindfulness meditation, exercise, calling a friend, knitting, solving a puzzle, for example) before you stumble on the strategy—or strategies—that work best for you. You'll find additional suggestions elsewhere in this chapter.

### Accept That the Situation You Are Facing Is Stressful

Accept the painful emotions and let them flow through you, reminding yourself that feelings come and feelings go and that you are not your feelings. This is more effective than trying to suppress painful emotions (a strategy that tends to result in the suppression of positive emotions as well as negative emotions) or dwelling on painful emotions (which ties up cognitive resources, leaving you less equipped to solve problems or to connect with other people).

### Rewrite Your Inner Monologue

Pay attention to the message in your head and replace any unkind or unhelpful messages with calming and affirming statements, like "I am doing the best that I can in a difficult situation." Learn how to recognize and steer clear of the following types of thinking traps, which can negatively affect your thinking, moods, and behavior:

- *All-or-nothing thinking:* "You always . . ." or "You never . . ."
- *Jumping to conclusions based on limited evidence:* "The doctor didn't return my phone call. Obviously, he doesn't care about our family."
- *Worst-case scenario thinking:* imagining the worst.
- *Emotional reasoning:* treating your feelings as objective fact and refusing to consider any evidence to the contrary.
- *Taking things personally.*
- *Telling yourself how you "should" act* and ignoring all other options.
- *Hostile attribution bias:* assuming the worst about other people's intentions.

For help in detecting errors in thinking that can make life more difficult, you may want to read *Mind over Mood, Second Edition: Change How You Feel by Changing the Way You Think* by Dennis Greenberger and Christine A. Padesky.

### Practice Positive Reappraisal

Positive reappraisal involves taking a more balanced approach to sizing up a difficult situation, as opposed to focusing entirely on the negative aspects. For example, instead of focusing on your feelings of fatigue, you might consider how coping with your child's mental illness has made you a stronger person. People who practice positive reappraisal experience less stress, a greater sense of well-being, more positive emotions, and fewer symptoms of depression. "It is almost never what happens that affects us over time, but the story we tell ourselves about what happens," explains Patricia A. Coughlin in her contribution to the book *Integrative Psychiatry*.

You might even try turning your thinking about stress on its head entirely—treating it as an opportunity for growth as opposed to something solely life-zapping—a point that Stanford University professor Kelly McGonigal makes in her book *The Upside of Stress: Why Stress Is Good for You and How to Get Good at It.* "Focus on what you are going to do with the energy, strength, and drive that stress gives you. Your body is providing you access to all your resources to help you rise to this challenge. Instead of taking a deep breath to calm down, take a deep breath to sense the energy that is available to you."

### Tame Your Emotions by Taking Action

Taking action toward solving a problem (even something as simple as making a phone call) engages the rational-logical part of your brain, which can help to reduce feelings of anxiety and sadness. "You bring about activation of the frontal cortex, which then inhibits the stress-inducing activity of the amygdala, thus resetting your mental equilibrium," explains Richard Restak in *Think Smart: A Neuroscientist's Prescription for Improving Your Brain's Performance.* "Taking action helps people feel less depressed, whereas inaction or passivity creates sad feelings," confirms John Arden in *Rewire Your Brain: Think Your Way to a Better Life.*

### Take Mini-Vacations from the Worry

Taking action is important, but there's nothing wrong with taking mini-vacations from the worry to give yourself a mental health break. You need and deserve a break—and your child needs and deserves a parent who is practicing good self-care. Because trying to suppress worries doesn't work particularly well (your brain has to waste valuable resources trying to push the worry away), a more effective strategy is to switch activities and get your brain busy thinking about something else for a little while. You might want to try going for a walk (see Chapter 9 for more about the benefits of exercise in managing stress), talking to a friend (see Chapter 12 for more about the benefits of tapping into support), reading a book, watching a movie, playing a game, working on a puzzle, engaging in a hobby or interest, or doing something nice for someone else (which can work really well in getting your mind off your own worries). Meg, whose son, Jayden, has been diagnosed with an anxiety disorder, has found relief in physical activity—dance. "Growing up, I danced. That was my creative outlet and how I expressed myself. So, every Thursday evening, I head to the dance studio and release my stress and tension the best way I know how: on the dance floor."

# Boosting Positive Emotion

It's easy to spiral into depression when you're coping with a stressful situation. In fact, when you're dealing with a stressful situation on an ongoing basis, you have to work hard at not becoming depressed.

One of the most powerful things you can do to stop the downward slide is to shift your default emotion from negative to positive. This means making a conscious effort to spend as much time in a positive mood as possible.

"Maximize the time that you spend in the emotional state that you want to be in so that it comes naturally to you," says Arden. "You want it to be your default mood. Do everything that you can do to promote the thoughts, perspective, and behaviors that kindle a positive mood."

Positive emotions don't just boost our mood, by the way. They improve our cognitive functioning too. Positive emotions signal safety to our brains, improving our attention, memory, and ability to learn.

So what are some things you can do to boost your mood, according to the psychological research?

### Train Your Brain to Be Able to Evoke Feelings of Happiness on Demand

Start out by listening to uplifting music while looking at images that evoke feelings of happiness for at least 70 seconds at a time. If you continue to use this technique with the same music and the same images, over time you'll be able to produce the same feeling of happiness in your brain, simply by thinking about the images—at least according to researchers at the University of Zurich.

### Savor Sweet Experiences

"Research indicates that savoring a moment of experience for at least 30 seconds strengthens the traces of neural firing in our memory," notes Linda Graham in her book *Bouncing Back: Rewiring Your Brain for Maximum Resilience and Well-Being.* And learning to savor sweet experiences makes them last, notes Coughlin in her contribution to the book *Integrative Psychiatry*: "Those who tend to savor sweetness and victories in life are happier and more satisfied than those for whom such experiences are fleeting. By consciously and intentionally sharing positive experiences, building strong memories of the peak moments in life, as well as celebrating the best of oneself, we can enhance well-being considerably." So take time to savor the truly amazing moments with your child and with others you love, so that you can draw on these positive memories in difficult times.

### Get an Oxytocin High

Don't overlook the power of oxytocin when it comes to helping you cope with stress. Connecting with—or even thinking about—someone who makes you feel loved, accepted, and safe releases this love-and-connection hormone into the brain and bloodstream, bringing cortisol levels and blood pressure down. Something as simple as looking at photos that remind you of happy times can give you the oxytocin boost you're craving.

### Make Plans to Do Something You Enjoy

It's tempting to put everything on hold when your child is struggling because your life feels out of control, but that's all the more reason to schedule activities you enjoy. You need and deserve a regular injection of positive emotion in your life. You may not feel like making the effort—it's easier to slip into a rut of inertia—but that's all the more reason to motivate yourself to do something pleasurable. As Sheri Van Dijk explains in her book *Calming the Emotional Storm*, "Especially when your mood is low or you have problems with anxiety or anger, you can't wait to feel like doing things. You often won't feel like doing an activity until after you've started doing it." Just don't expect your totally stressed-out brain to be able to come up with ideas for much-needed diversions. Take advantage of a time when you're not feeling stressed to the max and use this time to jot down a list of activities you enjoy. That way, the next time you're feeling too stressed to be creative, you can simply pull out your list and choose an activity. Realistically, you may find it works well to come up with separate lists for activities that can be enjoyed in almost no time at all (having a cup of tea, listening to your favorite song) and activities that require a bit more planning and commitment (having lunch with a friend). If you're having a hard time coming up with ideas for your list, ask a friend or family member to brainstorm with you.

### Master a New Skill

The sense of accomplishment we derive from learning something new helps us feel better about ourselves, improving our mood and leaving us less susceptible to the stress associated with difficult situations. Psychologist Mihaly Csikszentmihalyi has also discovered that we feel "happier, more cheerful, stronger, more active, more creative, more concentrated and more motivated" when we're engaged in a demanding and challenging activity.

## Maintain Your Sense of Optimism

"Optimism is often defined as an ability to maintain realistic hope and a sense of personal efficacy in relation to one's life goals," notes Coughlin. Optimists tend to focus on what they *can* control rather than what they *can't*, thereby reducing the amount of stress they experience.

## Foster Resilience

"Capacities for resilience—bouncing back when you're thrown off center—are evolutionarily hardwired into your brain, part of your birthright for coping with the stresses inherent in being alive and human," says Graham in *Bouncing Back*. We learn how to recover from, and even grow from, traumatic experiences by spending time with other resilient human beings. So, one of the best things you can do while your child is struggling is to line up plenty of support for yourself, by connecting with parent support groups and by reaching out to others in your life who truly care. (See Chapter 12 for more on this subject.)

## Foster Feelings of Gratitude

Intentionally focusing on feelings of gratitude reduces stress, enhances mental clarity, improves functioning of the autonomic nervous system, lowers blood pressure, and boosts your mood. It's also easy to do. Write down three things you're grateful for each day. Share gratitude reflections via social media. Or silently reflect on things you're grateful for throughout your day.

## Discover Your Purpose and Passion

It's easier to maintain enthusiasm for life and to bounce back from life's setbacks if you're clear about your purpose and passion. "Discovering your passion and finding a way to have that passion serve others is a key to creating a life that matters," notes Coughlin in *Integrative Psychiatry*. "Leading a purpose-driven life greatly enhances life satisfaction." Todd B. Kashdan and Joseph Ciarrochi make a similar point in their book *Mindfulness, Acceptance, and Positive Psychology*: "A purpose provides a foundation that allows a person to be more resilient to obstacles, stress, and strain. Persistence is easier with a life aim that resonates across time and context. It is easier to confront long-lasting difficult challenges with the knowledge that there is a larger mission in the background. Moving in the direction of a life aim can facilitate other elements of well-being such as life satisfaction, serenity, and mindfulness."

# Learning How to Relax

Relaxation techniques can help to ease your mind, relax your muscles, and leave you feeling centered and calm. They're particularly useful if you're worried, restless, having trouble sleeping, or struggling with anxiety or depression. Experiment with the different techniques until you find the ones that work best for you. And encourage your child to do the same.

### Relaxation Breathing

One of the simplest things we can do to help our brains and bodies relax is to switch to relaxation breathing: deep, slow, stomach-level breathing, rather than the fast, shallow, chest-level breathing we use when we're feeling stressed. To practice relaxation breathing, follow these steps:

1. Find a quiet, dimly lit, comfortable place where you can lie down.
2. Breathe in deeply so that your stomach fills with air. Then slowly exhale. (If you're trying to explain relaxation breathing to a child, ask her to pretend that she's filling and emptying a balloon in her stomach or trying to blow out the flame on an imaginary candle.)
3. As you continue to breathe in and breathe out slowly, notice your stomach rising and falling. If you place a hand on your stomach, you will be able to feel it rising as you breathe in and falling as you breathe out. Or try breathing in through your nose and out through your mouth—and, when you're breathing out through your mouth, pretend you are blowing through a bubble wand.
4. Try not to focus on anything but your breathing. You may find it helpful to focus on the word *breathe* as you breathe in and breathe out.
5. Repeat until you begin to feel relaxed or even sleepy.
6. Relax and then get up slowly when you are ready.

### Positive Visualization

Positive visualization involves transporting yourself to a world you've created in your own mind whenever you need a break from the stresses of the real world. To practice positive visualization, follow these steps:

1. Find a quiet, dimly lit, comfortable place where you can lie down.
2. Start your relaxation breathing.
3. Close your eyes and imagine a place where you feel safe and calm. Focus on what you are feeling and experiencing (sights, scents, sounds). Create a very detailed "movie" in your mind.

4. Play this movie in your mind until you feel the stress leaving your body.
5. Remind yourself that you can replay this movie whenever you need a break.
6. Relax, and then get up slowly when you are ready.

## Progressive Muscle Relaxation

Progressive muscle relaxation involves tensing and then relaxing each small muscle group in the body to encourage relaxation or to aid sleep. To practice progressive muscle relaxation, follow these steps:

1. Find a quiet, dimly lit, comfortable place where you can lie down.
2. Start your relaxation breathing.
3. Close your eyes and relax your entire body. Pretend that the muscles in your body are floppy, like noodles.
4. Start out by flexing the muscles in your feet for 5 seconds while keeping the rest of the muscles in your body relaxed. Relax for 15 seconds.
5. Proceed to flex the other muscle groups one by one (calves, thighs, hands, arms, stomach, chest, neck and shoulders, mouth, eyes, forehead), alternating with periods of relaxation.
6. Relax, breathe slowly and deeply, and imagine all of the tension leaving your body.
7. Get up slowly when you are ready.

NOTE: Your teenager may be more willing to try this technique when he is by himself, in which case he might find it helpful to read the progressive muscle relaxation instructions into an audio file on his computer or smartphone so that he can listen to the instructions rather than reading them while he tries to relax.

## Robot to Rag Doll

This is a fun one to share with your child, because the cues are so easy to remember.

1. Start out by making your body stiff, like a robot. (Or, if you prefer, think of the stiff-armed and stiff-legged movements of the poor old Tin Man in The Wizard of Oz.)
2. Then switch into rag-doll mode. Flop onto a soft surface like a mattress, allowing your arms and legs to go floppy, like noodles.

3. Note the difference between the two states—how you carry your body when you're tense like a robot or relaxed like a rag doll.

4. Remind yourself that you can let go of the tension that you're carrying—become more like a rag doll—whenever you feel yourself tensing up like a robot.

### Heavy and Warm

Try this relaxation exercise, which involves focusing on sensations of heaviness and warmth, with your child too.

1. Find a quiet, dimly lit, comfortable place where you can lie down.
2. Start your relaxation breathing.
3. Lying on your back, close your eyes and relax your entire body.
4. Focus on your right foot while telling yourself, "My right foot feels heavy." As you say this to yourself, imagine your foot sinking lower and lower and becoming heavier than the rest of your body. Repeat this phrase three times, imagining your foot becoming heavier and heavier.
5. Focus on your right foot while telling yourself, "My right foot feels warm." As you say this to yourself, imagine a very warm blanket on your foot. Repeat this phrase three times, imagining your foot becoming warmer and warmer.
6. Focus on your right foot while telling yourself, "My right foot feels heavy and warm." As you say this to yourself, imagine a warm, heavy blanket covering your foot. Repeat this phrase three times, imagining your foot getting heavier and warmer.
7. Repeat this series of exercises using your left foot, your stomach, your arms, and your head. If you have only a few minutes, just focus on relaxing one or two body parts.

## Other Mind and Body Practices

You might also be interested in looking into the stress-reduction benefits of other mind and body practices, including the following ones I've listed. Many of these techniques are used in therapy programs, so don't be surprised if you and your child encounter them as part of her treatment.

### Mindfulness Meditation

Mindfulness meditation focuses your attention on the present moment. Regular practice can leave you feeling calm and alert, improve your mood, increase feelings of compassion and empathy, reduce symptoms of stress, and lead to greater relationship satisfaction. "When you are being mindful, you are better able to see clearly what is happening in each moment of your life. As a result, you gain new insights into your experience, which greatly enhances your ability to tolerate difficult situations and to make wiser decisions," notes Phillip Moffitt in *The Best Buddhist Writing 2013*. Look online to find instructional videos and audio podcasts that will provide you with an introduction to mindfulness meditation. Or sign up for a mindfulness meditation workshop in your community. A growing number of mental health agencies are beginning to offer mindfulness meditation workshops as a treatment option.

### Massage Therapy

Massage therapy involves manipulating the soft tissues of the body for therapeutic purposes. It can help people of all ages relax and sleep better. It has also been demonstrated to help reduce stress levels in children and teenagers undergoing psychiatric treatment and to improve sleep and behavior in children with autism. And teenagers with ADHD who received massage therapy weekly for 1 month demonstrated improved moods and better classroom behavior (more time on task, less fidgeting, and less hyperactivity) when compared to other teenagers with ADHD who had been trained in relaxation techniques.

### Aromatherapy

Aromatherapy can also be an effective method of reducing stress and promoting relaxation. According to Kathi J. Kemper, author of *Mental Health, Naturally: The Family Guide to Holistic Care for a Healthy Mind and Body*, "Even very dilute concentrations of lavender aromas can significantly reduce levels of cortisol, a hormone linked to stress," while also improving the quality of sleep, while sage can "help clarify thinking and improve mood."

 **CAUTION:** Aromatherapy oils should be stored out of the reach of children, as many can be lethal if ingested.

### Acupuncture

While you might initially cringe at the idea of acupuncture—it involves having a trained practitioner stimulate specific pressure points on the body, most often by inserting thin needles through the skin—acupuncture is actually far less cringe-worthy than you might think. Fewer than 5% of people undergoing acupuncture treatment actually find acupuncture needles painful. That's good news for people seeking treatment for conditions like anxiety, depression, and insomnia. According to Kemper, "Acupuncture treatments . . . affect the activity and balance within the autonomic nervous system, generally increasing the sense of well-being and decreasing the fight-or-flight stress response."

### Biofeedback

Biofeedback is a technique that allows you to learn how to regulate your body's responses. It has been proven effective for promoting relaxation, reducing anxiety, improving mood, reducing the amount of time it takes to fall asleep, and enhancing attention and focus. Today's generation of biofeedback devices work with your home computer to gather information about your body's physiological responses (heart rate, skin temperature, perspiration rate, and so on) so that you can learn how to tune into and regulate these responses.

### Yoga

Yoga combines relaxation breathing and meditation. Even young children can benefit from this form of exercise, which promotes balance of the body and mind. It can help children feel a sense of control over their environment while providing much-needed calm during difficult situations. It also promotes better sleep, which leads to a happier, healthier child (to say nothing of a happier, healthier you).

Remember, putting in the effort to deal with your own stress and to find your own mental and emotional equilibrium is not selfish—it's a first step to helping the others in your family. If you're finding it difficult to bring your stress levels down on your own, don't be afraid to reach out for outside support, either from your child's pediatrician or other primary care provider, a counselor, or a parent support group. You don't have to deal with this on your own. Says Darlene, whose daughter Alicia struggled with an eating disorder throughout her teen years: "It's a sign of strength to seek help."

# 6

# Parents *Can*
# Make a Difference

So far, we've heard from parents that raising a child with a mental health or development challenge can be worrying, frightening, stressful, infuriating, and guilt-inducing. There are a lot of negative feelings that seem to come along for the ride, and none of them are helpful to the process.

In this chapter, we're going to be talking about parenting strategies that have proven helpful to other parents in the same situation—strategies that can help you dig yourself out of the emotional muck and get yourself back on solid ground. This discussion is all about building on the loving connection you already have with your child, being your child's voice, validating your child's emotions, creating a predictable environment, being a positive parent, and practicing what is known as mindful parenting. The goal is an even stronger parent–child relationship, a happier child, and a happier you.

> Your child really needs to know you are on this path together.
> **Alison, mother of Charlotte, who has been diagnosed with an anxiety disorder**

## Building on the Loving Attachment between You and Your Child

The most powerful tool in your parenting tool kit is the loving connection between you and your child.

As humans, we are wired for emotional connection with others. When our relationship connections are supportive, we feel comforted, and our brains become trained in such a way that we become capable of comforting ourselves. "Interactions with others—such as experiencing empathic, responsive parenting—instill a sense of safety and trust, a sense of importance and being loved, and a sense of competence and mastery that become your brain's first templates of resilience and serve as lifelong buffers from stress and trauma," explains Linda Graham in her book *Bouncing Back: Rewiring Your Brain for Maximum Resilience and Well-Being*.

The term *dyadic regulation* (which basically means two people connecting, communicating, and working at coordinating their emotional responses) is used to describe the process by which the brain of a calm and loving parent helps the brain of a crying baby soothe itself—how one person's nervous system is able to calm and regulate the nervous system of another person. That meeting of minds allows children to learn how to recognize and contain overwhelming feelings. Over time, the child comes to see himself as capable of adjusting his behavior to meet his own needs. We'll be talking more about this in the next chapter, but for now, all you need to know is that this foundation of love and trust is hardwired into our brains and plays a critical role in supporting mental health.

> The meeting of two personalities is like the contact of two chemical substances: if there is any reaction, both are transformed.
>
> **Carl Gustav Jung**

## Being Your Child's Voice

Sometimes one of the most powerful things you can do for a child who is struggling with feelings that seem overwhelming is to help her put those feelings into words. That way, she can experience the relief that comes from knowing she has been heard and understood.

"Dawson didn't have the ability to say what he really needed, so it was our job to do that for him," explains Mark, whose son has been diagnosed with reactive attachment disorder, an anxiety disorder, and a moderate developmental disability. "I make every decision with that in the back of my mind. He is 12 now and able to communicate so much better about what is going on and how he feels about things, so it's easier to make those decisions. But until your child can help you with that part, trust your gut and be that voice."

Lisa, whose daughter, Laura, is currently awaiting diagnosis, has also found that doing her best to be that voice has helped her relationship with her daughter. "On really bad days, I go and watch her when she's finally gone to sleep. Her face is at peace and I remember she's just a little kid who doesn't understand. She'll say to me sometimes, 'I don't know why it matters, but it does,' and that's my cue that she's not just being stubborn. Don't get me wrong—she got a double dose of stubborn too, but I've learned to hear what she can't say."

Resist the temptation to force conversations with your child. Learn to be comfortable with silence. Your child may need a moment to collect her thoughts before she speaks. Jumping in with advice or judgment may shut down the conversation before it even has a chance to get started.

Likewise, try not to jump to conclusions about what you think your child might be thinking or feeling. Test out those assumptions by checking them out with your child. Remind yourself that you are trying to be your child's voice, which means capturing his experience from his point of view ("I wonder if you are feeling frustrated because the teacher had to cancel gym class because of the fire drill, and that made it hard for you to settle down and do your work"). If your child or teenager responds with "No, that's not it at all! You just don't get it!" resist the temptation to become frustrated with your child—or yourself—and to shut down the conversation altogether. You may feel like you're playing emotional charades with your child as you try to make sense of a series of cryptic clues. The experience can be challenging and frustrating—you want so badly to get it right, but sometimes you simply can't find the right words. But it can also be incredibly rewarding when you manage to stumble across an insight that is helpful to you and your child.

To cope with your frustration in the moment, remind yourself that you're doing the best you can to understand, and he's doing the best he can to convey what happened from his own point of view. You may have to go back and forth a few times before you manage to pinpoint the source of his frustration and outrage and adequately translate those feelings into words ("You were upset because the teacher didn't seem to understand that canceling gym class was a big deal for you"). And there will be days when you simply aren't able to help your child voice those powerful feelings, despite your best efforts.

In situations like this, you may wish to move on to an emotional Plan B—a technique that is known as demonstrating affective attunement (mirroring the other person's emotions). Mirroring emotions (making a sad face yourself when your child is expressing sadness, for example) demonstrates to the child that his feelings have been acknowledged and understood. When a child feels understood, he feels reassured and cared for, and he is able to begin to calm himself down. At that point, you'll be better able to translate his experiences into words and to help him deal with the underlying issues. We use mirroring a lot with babies (imagine the sad face and voice you use to empathize with a baby who is crying) and younger children, but it is highly effective with older children and even teenagers too. It's a powerful and immediate way to telegraph emotional understanding and connectedness to your child.

## Validating Your Child's Emotions

Just as it takes some children a little longer to learn how to walk or to talk, it takes some children a little longer to learn how to regulate (recognize and manage) their emotions. One of the most effective strategies you can teach a child who is having angry outbursts, struggling with anxiety, or feeling overwhelmed by sad feelings is to reach out to other people for support. As Graham explains, reaching out for help involves "using the stability of other people's brains to stabilize our own."

When you encourage your child to connect with you emotionally, you're encouraging her to rely on the stability of your brain for help in regulating her emotions. You can do this by mirroring your child's feelings (through words, facial expressions, and body language) to show that you understand what she is trying to tell you. This helps to validate your child's feelings.

Validating your child's feeling is like a supercharged version of sympathizing with your child. It takes things one step further. You let your child know that what she is thinking and feeling makes sense (even if you don't happen to share that exact same perspective). You might tell your child, for example, that it makes sense to be afraid of thunder: everyone is afraid of sudden noises. Your goal is to encourage your child to accept her feelings rather than try to avoid them. Over time, this will help your child learn to accept and manage her emotions.

It's also an approach that works well in calming an upset child. Here's why. When your child is extremely upset, she won't be able to hear any rational arguments you are trying to make. This is because the part of her brain that gets fired up when she's extremely upset blocks the part of her brain that responds to logic and reason. (Think about how you felt the last time your computer crashed when you were working on something really important and a coworker decided to chime in with some unwanted tech tips.) She won't be able to process anything logical you're saying until she calms down—and the best way to get her to calm down is by validating her emotions so she feels heard. For example, "You are really disappointed that we didn't have time to stop at the library, the way we had planned. You were really looking forward to picking out some new books." At that point—once she feels heard—you can switch to the logic channel and start brainstorming solutions. Or the two of you can simply move on.

You'll want to stay calm while you're validating your child's feelings, because if you become upset, your child will pick up on your feelings and become more upset herself. You may find it helpful to repeat a calming phrase to yourself—something like "This too shall pass," "Just be kind," or "Breathe." If you're finding it difficult to remain calm in the face of powerful emotions from your child, ask yourself what your child needs from you right now and then try to act on that need. Maybe your child needs help managing emotions that are too big and too scary for her to handle on her own. Maybe she needs to feel reassured of her emotional connection to you. If you can focus on identifying and meeting your child's needs, you'll be less likely to get stuck dwelling on your own feelings of frustration.

There are added benefits to validating your child's feelings, as Karyn D. Hall and Melissa H. Cook note in their book *The Power of Validation: Arming Your Child Against Bullying, Peer Pressure, Addiction, Self-Harm, and Out-of-Control Emotions*: "Feeling heard and understood strengthens the bond and attachment they feel toward you. . . . A validated child is one who feels confident that she can express who she is and how she feels to her parents with complete acceptance without fear of judgment. . . . Children learn that they are accepted and loved, no matter what feelings or thoughts they have."

Validating your child's feelings also eliminates the pressure you might otherwise feel to fix your child's problems or to try to chase away any painful emotions. Children whose feelings are validated learn that they are capable of coping with their feelings, even the painful ones, and that feelings are temporary. They also learn that feelings are valuable sources of information—they serve as our emotional radar—which is why we don't want to drive our feelings underground. Every feeling is a valid feeling, and we can learn to recognize and manage those feelings in ways that work for, not against, us.

What's powerful about learning how to validate your child's feelings is the fact that you can validate what your child is feeling without necessarily having to agree with your child's behavior in a particular situation. You can let your child know that you understand why she decided to skip school without having to agree that cutting class was the best way to deal with her anxiety about an upcoming test. So you don't have to

> What I learned about reflective listening and validation— these powerful tools changed everything.
>
> **Kristina, mother of 18-year-old Clare, who has been diagnosed with bipolar disorder and generalized anxiety disorder and who also suffers from food sensitivities and irritable bowel syndrome**

worry that you're being too permissive. What you're doing is conveying your unconditional love and acceptance—and what a gift that is to a child who is struggling.

## Creating a Predictable Environment

Children thrive when they know what to expect on a day-to-day basis, when routines are predictable and the rules stay the same, no matter which adult is in charge. So one of the simplest things you can do to reduce your child's stress level—and, frankly, your own stress level—is to create a more predictable environment.

"When you have a child with intense emotions, everyday chaos feels more out of control and exacerbates the reactivity of your child," note Pat Harvey and Jeanine A. Penzo in their book *Parenting a Child Who Has Intense Emotions: Dialectical Behavior Therapy Skills to Help Your Child Regulate Emotional Outbursts and Aggressive Behaviors.*

"For Gabriel, it has always been important that we be consistent, organized, structured," says Laura, his mother. "We need to explain things to him well in advance. This has always helped with the Asperger's [Asperger syndrome is now referred to by the umbrella term *autism spectrum disorder* in DSM-5] and has helped to lessen his anxiety with the OCD as well. For example, he leaves for Scout camp in a couple of days and we're already completely packed. We've double-checked the kit list and we've labeled everything, because the thought of losing anything stresses him out completely. We've gone over various possible scenarios and how he can handle them. We have even printed out the menu for the week, put it in a page protector, and packed it for him so he'll know what he will be eating each day.

"In terms of our daily life, Gabriel's drawers in his room are labeled so he can put his clothes where they belong. We plan our meals a week at a time and I actually post these menus on a chalkboard we keep on the counter. We tend to eat dinner at the exact same time each day. We've developed a strategy for him to be organized at school. We have a schedule for the week that is posted on the refrigerator. I have shown Gabriel how to use the Reminders feature in his iPhone so that he doesn't have to worry that he will forget something. Being organized and structured has helped Gabriel tremendously."

Eliminating unnecessary clutter and reducing the amount of background noise in the home (for example, the television set that stays on from dawn to dusk, even if no one is actually watching, and the low-level buzz of fans and machinery) can also help to provide structure and promote calm. Some children become overstimulated if they encounter a lot of visual and auditory distractions. If this is a problem for your child, you might want to consider creating a quiet spot in your home where your child can retreat if he needs to regroup.

It's also a good idea to help your child anticipate and prepare for changes to the usual schedule or routine, whenever possible. And we also need to be prepared to help our children cope with the inevitable curveballs of life that we have no way of predicting or planning around. Cars break down. People are late. And plans fall apart. When this happens, we can help our children by validating their feelings about what has happened, coming up with a Plan B, and moving on. We can't protect our children from these types of disruptions and disappointments—nor would be want to. We would be robbing them of the opportunity to become more resilient. But, at the same time, we can recognize that these types of curveballs are difficult for them and support them as they work on developing their resiliency skills.

Being clear about behavioral expectations, and ensuring that all the key adults in a child's life share the same expectations, can also help to prevent meltdowns. Having parents with dissimilar parenting styles makes it more difficult for children to predict how their parents are going to react, which can leave children feeling helpless, anxious, and depressed. If you and your partner have very different parenting styles, or if the two of you are no longer parenting your child under the same roof, it is important to find a way to get your parenting more in sync for the benefit of your child. Some parents find it helpful to work with a couple therapist to resolve these issues. If you keep your child's needs at the forefront of the discussion, you'll find it easier to share information and brainstorm solutions—to set aside issues of ego and to focus on making life better for your child.

It's also important to reinforce the behavioral expectations that you set for your child. If you set limits but don't enforce them, those limits don't exist. That said, you still have to exercise some common sense—to combine the art with the science of parenting.

Susan, whose son Jacob struggles with anxiety, explains: "Boundaries have to be set. Even though they struggle with mental illness, they still need to know that there are rules for the family that need to be followed. Flexibility is key too. There are times when we have made plans to go out and my son is having a 'down' moment. We have to realize that we have to roll with it sometimes—to take the time he needs to work through this down moment and then move forward with the day." And, yes, it is possible to be consistent (by providing the type of structure that allows your child to thrive) and flexible (by letting go of the little things that don't matter quite as much) at the same time.

Andrew balances the need to set limits with his desire to practice kindness and generosity in his dealings with his son David, who has been diagnosed with schizophrenia. "Setting limits is constant and very important in our ongoing relationship. We've learned that it is important not to reinforce 'bad behavior' by sweeping things under the carpet and not dealing with them. If he becomes verbally aggressive or rude [when they are on the phone], we hang up. If he becomes too demanding, we don't grant his request. . . . We also try to practice kindness and generosity by buying David takeout food a couple of times a month (a favorite thing of his) and getting him some clothes as needed. We recently bought him a laptop when he showed interest in getting back to computer games. We try to support any interest in positive activity because it's so rare."

Like Christine, whose son, Will, has been diagnosed with severe ADHD and an anxiety disorder, you may find yourself rethinking your approach to discipline with a child who is struggling. She explains: "Most forms of discipline don't work well for Will. Yelling and timeouts terrify him. His anxiety disorder makes him very uncomfortable spending time alone, so a timeout in his room is like torture for him. We had to change our whole way of thinking and make a shift from 'discipline' to setting 'boundaries.' Instead of, 'No, you can't do that,' we now say, 'Why don't you try this instead?' We often redirect inappropriate behaviors in this way. This works best for us. Rewarding good choices also works well. More and more often, when Will gets worked up over something, he will choose to take a timeout in his room or in the backyard to calm himself down. When it's his choice, this is very effective for him."

Cat, who has two children struggling with mental illness, also supports a less punitive approach to discipline: "Punishment for mental illness–related behaviors adds a lot of stress to the family, and I haven't found it to be very productive." Kristina agrees: "The problem is, when your child is plagued with suicidal ideation, you lose a *lot* of parental leverage. When they don't even care about being alive, and maybe even feel pretty strong compulsions to end their life, they don't care about whether you suspend video game or Internet privileges. They just sink deeper into despair when even those sole remaining pleasures have been lost."

Here's the thing: Punishment assumes that a child is capable of making different and better choices—and sometimes that simply isn't the case for a child who is struggling. "It's

> It is so important to understand what will work and won't work with a child who has FASD [fetal alcohol syndrome disorder]. And it's not a matter of the child not wanting to comply. It's a case of the child not being able to comply. Punishment doesn't work and sticker charts don't work either.
>
> **Linda, mother of Jesse, who lives with FASD**

not your child choosing to act badly. Something's gone haywire," says Liza Long, author of *The Price of Silence*. And, as psychology professor Stuart Shanker has noted, a child who is under considerable stress is not going to be able to regulate his emotions and behavior very effectively—and punishing that child will only exacerbate his or her difficulties with self-control.

So, in other words, looking for alternatives to punitive forms of discipline with a child who is struggling doesn't merely lead to a warmer and happier relationship between you and your child; it also increases the likelihood of your child being able to manage his behavior more appropriately. It's the ultimate parenting win–win.

## Being a Positive Parent

Are you a glass-half-empty kind of person? Many of us are. In fact, our brains are hardwired to see the dark side of everything. "Evolutionarily and culturally, we are hardwired and conditioned to look first for what's wrong, what's negative, and what's potentially dangerous in any situation," explains Graham in *Bouncing Back*.

While this negativity bias may be useful when it comes to preventing us from becoming some predator's next meal, it can take its toll on our personal relationships. "Because of the brain's negativity bias, we can become, and remain, quite negative about other people and our relationships with them," says Graham.

That explains a lot, now, doesn't it? But wait! It gets worse! This negativity bias can take on a life of its own when your family is going through a rough time.

A study published in a 2012 issue of *European Child & Adolescent Psychiatry* noted that children who have been diagnosed with mental illness tend to see their parents as behaving negatively toward themselves and their siblings, despite the fact that their healthier siblings describe their parents as behaving *positively* toward themselves and their siblings.

Meanwhile, parents of teenagers who are struggling with depression tend to make more negative comments about their teenagers' behavior than parents of teenagers who are not depressed. "The challenges and frustrations of parenting an adolescent with depression may, over time, result in more automatic and less sensitive parental causal explanations for the adolescent's behavior," noted a group of researchers from the Oregon Research Institute and the University of British Columbia in a study published in 2012 in the *Journal of Family Psychology*.

One of the most powerful things you can do to support a child who is struggling with mental health or development challenges is to try to break free of this cycle of negativity. Not only will you feel better, you will be able to come up with better solutions to the problems facing your family. As Barry Trute and colleagues noted in a study published in the *Journal of Child and Family Studies*, "While negative emotions limit attention to solve challenges, and deplete energy to deal with problems at hand, positive emotions broaden the scope of thinking and widen the boundaries of problem solving. Positivity thus builds personal and relational resources in parents as they respond to ongoing family challenges and seek their solution."

A powerful way to up the amount of positivity in your life is by shaking up your thinking about your child. Instead of focusing on the things you wish you could change about your child (the glass half empty), begin to focus on the things you love and admire about your child (the glass half full). And be sure to comment on the types of behaviors you are noticing so your child benefits from some positive reinforcement too. Commenting on specific behaviors in the moment tends to work particularly well. For example, you might say to your child, "I see how patient you are being with your sister today—even when she is being really frustrating. That takes a lot of self-control!" You might want to keep track of these observations in the "Strengths" section of the binder you have created for your child (see Chapter 4).

> **NOTE:** You'll find it easier to identify your child's strengths if you have appropriate expectations for your child. It's a good idea to remind yourself that children—like adults—are works in progress. They are still learning and growing, and much of that growing involves learning how to manage their thoughts, feelings, and behaviors more effectively. You can't (or shouldn't) expect a 6-year-old to have the emotional maturity of an adult.

As your attitude toward your child begins to shift, you are likely to notice a corresponding change in your behavior too. You might even notice a difference in your child's behavior over time. When parents are positive and supportive, children are more likely to listen and find it easier to control their emotions and behaviors.

## Fostering Confidence in Your Child

Stanford University psychology professor Carol S. Dweck has devoted much of her career to studying self-theories: how people's beliefs about themselves create psychological worlds that motivate thoughts, feelings, and behavior. She has focused particular attention on how children develop self-theories (and how parents' best intentions to help children feel good about themselves sometimes backfire).

"Parents think they can hand children permanent confidence—like a gift—by praising their brains and talent," she explains in her book *Mindset: The New Psychology of Success*. "It doesn't work, and in fact has the opposite effect. It makes children doubt themselves as soon as anything is hard or anything goes wrong. If parents want to give their children a gift, the best thing they can do is to teach their children to love challenges, be intrigued by mistakes, enjoy effort, and keep on learning. That way, children don't have to be slaves of praise. They will have a lifelong way to build and repair their own confidence."

Children who seek validation through achievement do just fine . . . until they make a mistake. Even a small misstep can undermine their sense of self-worth, leaving them feeling anxious and unwilling to tackle new challenges. Less vulnerable children, on the other hand, recognize that making a mistake is not the end of the world, because their self-worth doesn't depend on being right all the time.

## Looking for Little Ways to Make Things Better

"Don't underestimate the power that the practical stuff can have," says Cheyenne, whose daughter, Keisha, has been diagnosed with ADHD and anxiety. You may not be able to change who your kid is—the reactions or the illnesses—but you can modify the environment to make life easier for the child and for you. That means asking yourself what would help to make things better in a situation that is difficult for your child. "Relax your rules and rethink your ideas about the way things should be," she suggests. "I used to say I'd never let my kids wear headphones everywhere. Guess what? She wears headphones everywhere. Who cares? She can put them on and it blocks the whole world out"—something that allows Keisha to cope at times when the world might otherwise feel overwhelming.

## Practicing Mindful Parenting

Mindfulness can refer to two different but related things. It can refer to a conscious meditation practice (a proven method of stress release—mindfulness meditation—that we touched on in the previous chapter). And it can refer to heightening your awareness when approaching a particular task. As Sheri Van Dijk explains in her book *Calming the Emotional Storm*,

"Anything you do, you can do mindfully . . . if you focus your full attention on that activity, in the present moment, with acceptance."

> Mindfulness means paying attention in a particular way; on purpose, in the present moment, and nonjudgmentally.
> **Jon Kabat-Zinn, founder of the Stress Reduction Clinic at the University of Massachusetts Medical School**

The benefits of taking a mindful approach are pretty obvious. Instead of reacting in the moment, you're able to pause long enough to make conscious and deliberate choices about your parenting—an approach that allows you to make better decisions with fewer regrets. You're more accepting and less judgmental of yourself and your child, which allows you to make better parenting decisions and to feel better about yourself as a parent. And you're able to focus on your progress toward big-picture parenting goals that are in sync with your values and reflect the relationship you hope to have with your child over a lifetime. It's a powerful approach to parenting.

In an article published in the *Clinical Child and Family Psychology Review*, Larissa G. Duncan, J. Douglas Coatsworth, and Mark T. Greenberg have identified five aspects of mindful parenting that enhance the parent–child relationship:

- Listening with full attention
- Practicing nonjudgmental acceptance of yourself and your child
- Being aware of your emotions and your child's emotions in the moment
- Being able to control your own emotions in the moment
- Having compassion for yourself and your child

*Listening with full attention* means really tuning in to what your child is saying, both through her words and her tone of voice and through her facial expressions and body language. Your goal is to figure out what your child is trying to tell you and what she needs from you.

*Nonjudgmental acceptance of yourself and your child* is also at the heart of mindful parenting. "Mindful parenting involves a nonjudgmental acceptance of the traits, attributes, and behaviors of self and child," write Duncan, Coatsworth, and Greenberg. This kind of no-strings-attached acceptance can be incredibly freeing, particularly for children. How your child sees himself is affected in large part by the language you use to describe him. If you can teach yourself to use descriptive (*effective* or *ineffective*, *helpful* or *unhelpful*, *healthy* or *unhealthy*) rather than judgmental language (*good* or *bad*), your child is less likely to feel judged, and he will find it easier to tease out the connections between his behavior, your reaction, and how he is feeling. He is also more likely to feel connected to you. And while feeling judged may cause him to lose confidence in his ability to change his behavior, feeling loved will reduce his anxiety and give him the confidence and the motivation to continue to try changing the behaviors that aren't working for him.

Don't expect to be able to avoid judgmental language right away: this skill takes practice. As Van Dijk notes, "At first, you'll notice your judgments only after you've made them. As you continue practicing, however, you'll notice them as you're making them—before you say them out loud and they form in your head—until gradually, you'll find you're able to form nonjudgmental statements naturally before a judgment arises within you."

*Being aware of your emotions and your child's emotions in the moment* means "paying attention with openness, curiosity, and flexibility," to borrow a phrase from Todd B. Kashdan and Joseph Ciarrochi, coauthors of *Mindfulness, Acceptance, and Positive Psychology: The Seven Foundations of Well-Being.* Because you are remaining calm and reflective, you are able to make conscious choices about how to respond. You are also able to increase your effectiveness as a parent. "[Mindful parents] reflect on the positive and negative affect that they and their child experience and express during parenting interactions and how their moods influence one another. These activities also help parents identify situations . . . in which they are more likely to experience uncomfortable emotions that can escalate into interactions filled with angry and hurtful words and actions," note Duncan, Coatsworth, and Greenberg.

> True others are those who can see and reflect our true self back to us when we have forgotten, or perhaps have never known, who we truly are. They remember our best self when we are mired in our worst self and accept without judgment all of who we are.
> **Linda Graham,**
> *Bouncing Back: Rewiring Your Brain for Maximum Resilience and Well-Being*

*Being able to control your own emotions in the moment* means making a conscious choice to exhibit parenting behavior that is in sync with your parenting values and goals. "Mindful parenting does not imply that the impulse to display negative affect, anger, or hostility is not felt, but mindful parenting involves pausing before reacting in parenting interactions in order to exercise greater self-regulation and choice in the selection of parenting practices," Duncan, Coatsworth, and Greenberg explain. What's more, by showing your child how to label, express, and talk about feelings, you can help your child learn how to manage her emotions more effectively. (Note: We'll be returning to this topic in Chapter 7.)

> The biggest challenge for me was getting past taking it personally. It took me a very long time to accept that he had a mental illness and he was not deliberately targeting us. This was how his brain was wired and his way of communicating that illness. Once we were able to accept that, we were able to learn to react in ways that were not emotionally charged. Until we learned to do this, everything was in crisis mode. Now we are stronger than ever as a couple and Dawson has learned how to communicate how he is feeling as well.
>
> **Mark, father of Dawson**

*Having compassion for yourself and your child* means recognizing that you and your child are each doing the best you can. It means relying on gentle encouragement rather than harsh judgment to motivate yourself and your child. It also means being kind to yourself and your child when you fall short of your own or one another's expectations. It means forgiving and moving on.

"We're hardwired to need compassion when we're feeling threatened in some way," explains Allison Kelly, an assistant professor of psychology at the University of Waterloo in Ontario, Canada. "And yet those who have more sensitive threat systems have a difficult time generating compassion for themselves and accessing compassion from other people." Treating your child with compassion helps to soothe him. It also teaches him that he can reach out to others for support when he is feeling uncertain or scared. And by treating him with compassion, you will be encouraging him to extend the same kindness to himself.

## Moving Forward

Psychologist Carl Rogers once said, "The curious paradox is that when I accept myself just as I am, then I can change." For this reason, one of the most powerful gifts you can give to your child is the gift of self-acceptance. Feeling lovable and worthy no matter what makes change and growth possible.

You can help your child reach this state of self-acceptance by using some of the techniques described earlier: voicing his feelings when he can't express them, validating his emotions, creating a predictable environment and setting constructive boundaries, making sure that parenting is consistent, being positive, and practicing mindful parenting. If you are looking for support as you embark on this journey, you may wish to consider the following strategies.

### Join a Parent Support Group

If you are already a member of a parent support group, you might want to try raising some of these subjects with other parents there. It could lead to some helpful discussions or tried-and-true tips from parents in the same boat.

### Look into Parenting Resources

You might find help from parenting resources (books, workshops, groups) that expose you to new ideas about parenting—ideally ideas that have worked for other parents who have faced parenting challenges similar to your own. Of course, you'll want to keep doing the part of parenting that comes naturally: loving your child, no matter what.

### Consider Family, Individual, or Couple Therapy

You might find support here for discussions about family practices, boundary setting, and finding a consistent parenting style. How we parent is often a function of how we ourselves were parented, and if you and your parenting partner are having trouble reaching a consensus on important issues, it might be helpful to find someone who can help you explore the origins of your attitudes and habits.

"Having the therapist teach us some new approaches was a light-bulb moment," says Jennifer. "My focus was so much on getting Jess treatment that I never stepped back far enough to see that it was actually crucial for me and her father to learn some new skills. We feel so much more equipped to handle the transition to adulthood now. And we know this therapist has our back—she'll be there if we need more guidance or run into bumps in the road. I can't express how good that feels."

# 7

# Calming the Raging Storm

I used to wear long sleeves to cover the bite marks and bruises after Janine had a bad day. I would fall into bed exhausted at night with a sense of hopelessness.

**Mary, mother of Janine, who has a mild intellectual disability and is on the autism spectrum, and Fiona, who has been diagnosed with bipolar disorder**

Psychologists use the term *emotional regulation* to describe what you and I tend to think of as emotional control—the ability to monitor, evaluate, and adjust our emotions to make them best meet our needs at any given time.

The ability to regulate emotions is acquired over a period of years, and it doesn't come easily or naturally to every child. Some children inherit genes that increase the likelihood that they will struggle with anxiety, irritability, depression, and impulsivity; some are temperamentally wired to experience emotions more intensely than other children; and some may have difficulty processing emotions as a result of cognitive challenges.

When a child has difficulty regulating his emotions (a typical struggle for a child with ADHD or an autism spectrum disorder, for example), he is likely to struggle at school, in friendships, and at home. He may blurt out answers in class rather than wait his turn, annoying the teacher and his classmates. He may find it difficult to understand the unwritten rules of friendship, resulting in painful social blunders or an unwillingness to risk rejection at all. Or he may find it difficult to cope with change, resulting in angry outbursts.

If difficulty with emotional regulation is an issue for your child, there are a number of strategies you can use to help him learn how to predict and manage the situations that are causing the most distress. These are the types of strategies we're going to be discussing in the last part of this chapter—strategies that other parents have found helpful in reducing the amount of conflict and chaos in their children's lives.

But before a child can learn how to manage his emotions, he needs to be able to speak the language of emotions. That's why we're going to start out by talking about emotional literacy.

## Raising an Emotionally Literate Child

To thrive in the world, kids need to be emotionally literate—to be able to understand and speak frankly about emotions. They need to be able to connect the feelings associated with various types of emotions with the names for those emotions, so that they'll be able to talk about their feelings with others. They also need to understand the unwritten rules that come into play as we deal with our emotions—things like when and how to share emotions and with whom.

What we want to do is to give our kids—particularly kids who are struggling—a sense of mastery and control over their emotions, to leave them with the confidence that they can tackle their feelings head-on and use them as springboards to action. What we don't want is for our children to be afraid of their emotions, to try to avoid them or push them away because they feel too overwhelming.

Being emotionally literate (which is sometimes described as being emotionally intelligent) leads to greater happiness and life satisfaction—even improved physical health and increased longevity.

So what do kids need to know about emotions?

Quite a lot, actually.

Here's what they need to know.

• *People express feelings in a variety of different ways* (words, body language, facial expressions, sounds). What's more, the same emotion can be expressed in dramatically different ways by different people. For example, some people become very fidgety when they're anxious, while others fall asleep.

• *People can mask their emotions.* Sometimes it doesn't make sense to broadcast your emotions to the world, so you might decide to keep your feelings to yourself.

• *Emotions can be triggered by external circumstances (things outside us) and internal circumstances (things within us).* It's important to be aware of what's causing (triggering) emotions because emotions affect how we feel, what we think, and sometimes how we act too.

• *Emotions come in different intensities, like salsas.* They can range from mild to super-intense. Paying attention to the intensity of emotions allows people to choose a coping strategy that reflects how strongly they're feeling about something (for example, you might take a break from a very frustrating task but continue to plug away at a task that is only mildly frustrating). You can give your child practice in tuning in to the intensity of emotions by playing a game of emotional charades or by acting out emotions with hand puppets. Portray an emotion using gestures, body language, facial expressions, and sounds but no words. Ask your child to try to figure out which emotion it is that you're trying to portray and how intensely you are feeling that emotion. Are you a little bit excited or over-the-moon excited? Are you a little bit scared or terrified? Then give your child a turn at acting out emotions too.

• *The intensity of emotions can increase or decrease as circumstances change.* If you're having a bad day and something else happens to make it even worse, your feeling of frustration is likely to zoom even higher. But if a friend leaves a nice note on your desk, that feeling of frustration might disappear altogether. Likewise, the intensity of emotion associated with a particular event can change over time. You might be really upset today about getting a stain on your favorite sweater, but you are unlikely to be thinking about what happened a week from now (unless, of course, you really, really liked that sweater).

• *It is possible to experience more than one emotion at the same time.* You can be both excited and anxious about the first day at a new school, for example. Imagine putting on layers of emotion, like you might put on layers of clothing. Sometimes those layers clash and sometimes they work reasonably well together. It's the same way with emotions.

• *Everyone needs to work at regulating their emotions.* It's a skill that we develop through practice over time. And it's as much about boosting positive emotion as it is about bringing down levels of negative emotion. In other words, it's not enough to learn how to calm yourself when you're feeling angry; you also need to learn how to boost your mood when you're feeling blue.

Emotional regulation lays the groundwork for other areas of self-regulation, including regulating attention. As Shanker notes in his book

*Calm, Alert, and Learning: Classroom Strategies for Self-Regulation,* "If a child is depressed, frightened, anxious, angry, frustrated, or ashamed, that child will find it very difficult, if not impossible, to concentrate. Conversely, the calmer, happier, safer, and more curious, confident, and interested the child, the better that child will learn."

And, as the work of Oregon State University developmental psychologist Megan McClelland, coauthor of *Stop, Think, Act: Integrating Self-Regulation in the Early Childhood Classroom,* has demonstrated, strong self-regulation skills during the preschool years predict success in college-age students: "We found that kids who were rated as being really strong on being able to pay attention and to persist on difficult tasks when they were four years old had 50% greater odds of finishing college by the time they were 25," she notes. What's key is the delay of gratification—a skill you can help your child to develop. She suggests having children tackle tasks like puzzles that they find really challenging (so that they can work on focus and persistence—two skills that are key in self-regulation), and playing games in which the rules change as you play (so that they have to pay attention and then switch strategies—an act of mental gymnastics that helps kids work on another all-important skill: cognitive flexibility).

## What You Can Do

As a parent, you have a huge role to play in helping your child become emotionally literate, both by modeling healthy coping and self-regulation skills and by making emotion a subject of day-to-day conversation in your home.

### Look for Opportunities to Discuss Emotions with Your Child

Talk about how various characters handle certain emotionally charged situations in movies or TV shows you watch together or in books you read. Ask:

- What might have triggered their reactions?
- Did their reactions achieve the desired results?
- What other options might they have considered for handling their emotions?

Be sure to give your child the opportunity to see how you tackle the tough emotional stuff in real life. If you're feeling really frustrated because your computer just crashed for the third time while you were trying to pay a bill online, let your child hear you saying to yourself, "I think I need to take a break before I work on this again." Then get up and fold the laundry for a while. Or model effective problem-solving skills for your child by saying "Something keeps causing my browser to crash. I think I'd better reboot the computer before I do any more online banking."

If you happen to blow it (you become irate instead of modeling the calm behavior you had planned to exhibit), simply take a couple of deep breaths and let your child see you succeed at regaining control, albeit a little belatedly. You might not have gotten it on Take 1, but you persevered and got it on Take 2. You might also share a comment that will make the process even more explicit for your child. "Getting mad didn't fix my computer, so I'm trying something else: calming myself down. That way, I can start thinking about ways I can actually solve this problem. My brain doesn't do a very good job of solving problems when I'm angry or upset. Once I calm down, I'll be able to think a lot more clearly and I'll be able to figure out what to do next. I think I need a break. Would you like to go for a walk around the block with me?"

### Help Your Child Make Sense of Her Own Emotional Experiences by Accepting and Validating Her Emotions

This is something we talked about in Chapter 6. It's particularly important to remember to validate your child's negative emotions because that can help prevent those emotions from spiraling out of control. As researchers Nancy Eisenberg, Tracy L. Spinrad, and Natalie D. Eggum noted in a 2010 article in the *Annual Review of Clinical Psychology*, "Parental reactions to children's negative emotions provide children with valuable information about the experience and expression of emotions. Supportive responses and emotion coaching may help children reduce their negative emotions, contribute to children's abilities to understand emotions, or directly teach ways to deal with emotions in the future." A nonsupportive reaction, on the other hand, can trigger more negative emotion in your child, causing the situation to escalate.

Here's something else you need to know: A child who has difficulty regulating his emotions elicits more negative responses from his parents than a child who is more fully in control of his emotions. The same is true with other adults he interacts with, like teachers and coaches, as well as his peers. The negative emotion meets a negative response, reinforcing the child's negative emotion—and this cycle repeats.

But here you can make a difference. You can help to end the cycle by responding to your child in more positive ways, which will, over time, begin to shift the way in which your child responds to you. And as he begins to respond to you in new, more adaptive ways, his brain will begin to recognize this as his new normal. What's more, his emotional set-point will shift from negative to positive territory, and he will begin to elicit more positive responses from other people in his life as well.

You can help this process along by teaching your child strategies for increasing the amount of positive emotion he experiences—a topic we covered at length back in Chapter 5. And while you're helping him dial up the amount of positive emotion in his life by tapping into some of those strategies, you can also help him dial down the amount of anger and anxiety he is experiencing.

## Handling Angry Outbursts

Anger performs an essential function in our lives, letting us know when our personal boundaries have been violated and revving up our brains and our bodies for action.

The secret to making anger work for us, not against us, is to learn how to prevent feelings of anger from causing us to act in ways we might regret later. It's not a new problem. In fact, the Greek philosopher Aristotle had this to say on the subject over 2,000 years ago: "Anybody can become angry—that is easy. But to be angry with the right person and to the right degree and at the right time and for the right purpose, and in the right way—that is not within everybody's power and is not easy."

So what can you do to help a child who is finding it difficult to manage angry feelings, who responds intensely, or who reacts impulsively when faced with this particular emotion?

### Identify the Triggers

Start out by trying to figure out which types of situations are most likely to cause problems for your child. If you can identify your child's triggers, you're one step closer to being able to help her learn how to avoid or manage these types of situations.

So, what exactly is a trigger?

"The trigger for your child is anything that causes or leads to an intense emotional response," explain Pat Harvey and Jeanine A. Penzo, authors of *Parenting a Child Who Has Intense Emotions: Dialectical Behavior Therapy Skills to Help Your Child Regulate Emotional Outbursts and Aggressive Behaviors*. "No behavior occurs in isolation. The trigger may be something in the environment, or it may be something going on inside your child, like a thought or a feeling." For example, your child might have a tendency to assume the worst of other people—a thought pattern that may not reflect the reality of the situation, but one that can trigger reactions nonetheless. She might react with extreme anger at a perceived slight that wasn't actually a slight at all, or she might break off friendships at the first hint that someone might hurt or disappoint her. Likewise, she may have woken up feeling edgy and irritated today—the result of a restless night's sleep—causing her to react more strongly or negatively than you might expect or than might be considered appropriate.

### Problem-Solve the Triggers

In their book *Treating Explosive Kids: The Collaborative Problem-Solving Approach*, Ross W. Greene and J. Stuart Ablon recommend thinking of triggers as "problems that have yet to be solved"—by you, the parent, in collaboration with your child. After all, the easiest—and least stressful—way to deal with triggers is to help your child avoid becoming triggered in the first place. It certainly beats having to manage and deal with the fallout from an angry outburst.

Try to avoid situations that your child can't handle right now. You won't have to avoid these situations forever, but you'll save yourself and your child a lot of grief if you minimize the number of times you subject her—and yourself—to unnecessary frustration. You want your child to experience a series of successes so that she develops a sense of competence and mastery, a feeling that she can cope with whatever life tosses his way. The best way to help that happen is to set limits on the challenges she has to face at any given time and then gradually expose her to more and greater challenges. What doesn't help is to set her up for almost certain failure by forcing her to deal with challenges that are simply too much for her to deal with right now. The trick here is to learn how to walk the line between overchallenging and underchallenging her. It's not helpful (or possible) to shield her from all possible frustrations.

Once you have identified a situation that tends to trigger an angry outburst in your child (your child doesn't like it when you remind him to brush his teeth, for example), attempt to define the problem (your child needs to brush his teeth but doesn't like it when you remind him about it) and invite your child to work with you to find some possible solutions (would he like to set up an electronic reminder on the family computer to remind himself about brushing his teeth?). This is the collaborative problem-solving approach that Greene and Ablon recommend. What works is finding a solution that is effective for both you and your child. What doesn't work is trying to simply impose a solution that you consider to be acceptable; your child may reject and rebel against your solution, which will trigger even more feelings of anger. By coming up with a solution together, you are respecting your child's right to be involved in making decisions about his own life, while also recognizing the value of the life experience that you, as his parent, bring to the table. This process has the potential to build on the parent–child bond by encouraging the two of you to work together in achieving a mutual goal: finding creative solutions to the problem of triggers. So, ask your child what would make his life easier and how you can help, and let the creative problem solving begin. You'll find it works best if you address one trigger at a time, giving top priority to situations that will make the greatest difference in terms of improving life for your child, yourself, and your family. At the same time, look for opportunities to reduce your child's overall stress level. (You may want to give him a pass on keeping his room tidy for now.) A child who is less stressed overall is better able to manage feelings of anger.

### Help Your Child Be Body Smart

You can teach your child to recognize the way her body feels when she is starting to become angry. She is likely to notice that her heart starts beating faster, she begins to breathe more rapidly, and her body begins to feel tense—as though it wants to spring into action. This is because anger—like anxiety—triggers a fight-or-flight reaction.

### Help Your Child Learn to Put the Brakes On

Your child can learn to understand that acting on impulse when we're angry might lead to consequences we regret later. We need to put the brakes on long enough to consider our options before we act. To help with this, encourage your child to pay attention to how quickly he is becoming angry and just how angry he is feeling. (Some children find it helpful to rate their feelings of anger on a scale of 1 to 5 or to think of rising anger in terms of shades of yellow, orange, and then red.) Then help your child figure out ways he can deal with his rising anger before it reaches the danger zone, when it is much more difficult to control.

> Teach children how to replace "hot thoughts" with "cool thoughts." Hot thoughts are immediate. They encourage children to act impulsively. Cool thoughts come after taking a deep breath. They help children decide on the best way to handle a situation or solve a problem.
>
> **Susan E. Craig, *Reaching and Teaching Children Who Hurt: Strategies for Your Classroom***

Your child might want to experiment with the following types of solutions.

- Take a break from the situation.
- Think about something other than what's making him angry.
- Release anger in safe ways (such as through exercise).
- Let some things go (especially "the small stuff").
- Recognize inaccurate and unproductive patterns of thinking that are only serving to fuel anger (thought patterns that can be shifted through CBT; see Chapter 3).
- Work on any skills deficits that could be making it more difficult to manage those feelings of anger (see the chart on pages 130–132 and also Chapter 5 for additional stress management and coping strategies).

### Help Your Child Understand That Feelings Sometimes Come in Disguises

For example, sometimes people react with anger when they are experiencing other emotions they don't know how to manage, like anxiety, sadness, or shame. Encourage your child to ask herself a question like "Am I just feeling angry, or am I feeling something else too?" (like maybe frustration, embarrassment, or anxiety) so that she can pinpoint exactly what she's feeling and deal with any underlying emotions. See the discussion on teaching children about emotional literacy earlier in this chapter and consult Appendix B for links to some helpful online resources.

### Recognize That Your Child Might Need Additional Help

Sometimes a child doesn't have the ability to manage strong feelings like anger, anxiety, and sadness on her own. And yet this is what we are asking a child to do when she is sent to timeout or when we ask an older child or teenager to take a break from a situation until he has his feelings under control. Debra Andrews and William Mahoney, coeditors of *Children with School Problems: A Physician's Manual*, explain: "Sometimes it works well for child and parent to go to separate areas of the house so that the child can cool down. But some children, such as those with autism, need an opportunity to co-regulate [regulate their emotions with help from someone else] with a caregiver before they can self-regulate on their own. During this 'time-in' (as opposed to timeout) with a parent, the child could be encouraged to release energy (jumping, bouncing on a therapy ball). Then the caregiver can validate [the] child's emotions. This time together can help to nurture the parent–child relationship while helping the child to recover from stress and regain emotional balance."

As your child becomes calmer, you can help him gain insights from what has happened. Review together the incident that triggered the emotions. Encourage your child to describe what happened in his own words, from his own point of view, listing all the steps that led to the conflict or problem. At this point you simply want to listen as your child describes what happened and validate the feelings he experienced as the situation played out. Once your child has had a chance to be heard, you can gently suggest alternatives to his thinking (Did he jump to any mistaken conclusions about someone else's intentions that might have caused the situation to escalate?) and his behavior (What might he have done differently to change the outcome of the situation?). You can also talk about ways to prevent similar conflicts from arising in the future and about how to repair any damage resulting from the current conflict.

You might also want to help your child develop his decision-making skills by modeling these skills yourself and talking to him about what's involved in making good decisions (for example, how we tend to make better decisions when we're not tired or stressed out and when we remember to take other people's perspectives into account as well as our own). Just understand that it takes time for children to acquire these skills—and some kids a little longer than others. "'Good' decision-making is not hardwired," explains Joshua Weller, assistant professor of psychology at Oregon State University. "It involves skills that can be learned, just like you can learn other types of critical-thinking skills. But it takes time, practice, and effort."

### Recognize When You Need Support

While there is much you can do to help your child yourself, it's also important to know when you and your child might benefit from outside help: for example, if you're feeling as if you're running out of options, or if the situation has become intolerable for you and your child. "Some children may react to requests and simple changes and transitions with extreme inflexibility and aggression," note Andrews and Mahoney. "Such children generally do not respond as well to standard [discipline] strategies, and consequences may actually heighten their emotional arousal. Many children with autism spectrum disorders, sensory processing issues, or anxiety fall into this category. These families will likely need the help of a mental health therapist and sometimes a physician (child psychiatrist, pediatrician, developmental pediatrician) for medication. Managing these explosive outbursts requires investigating and treating the underlying cognitive and regulatory causes."

## Helping Your Child Manage Feelings of Anxiety

"If you are the parent or caregiver of an anxious child, you know what it feels like to be held hostage. So does your child," says Dawn Huebner in the introduction to her book *What to Do When You Worry Too Much*. "Children who worry too much are held captive by their fears. They go to great lengths to avoid frightening situations, and ask the same anxiety-based questions over and over again. Yet the answers give them virtually no relief."

If your child struggles with anxiety, it can be exhausting to be the person your child turns to for reassurance whenever she is feeling anxious or unsure. You may find yourself trying to act as the buffer between her and an ever-increasing number of situations that she finds too scary or too painful to tolerate—an unenviable position for anyone.

It's not as if you want to chase all of your child's anxious feelings away (if that were even possible). After all, she came hardwired to experience feelings of anxiety as a matter of survival. In situations involving real danger, you want her body to alert her to an impending threat and to tell her that it's time to switch into action mode. Anxiety becomes a problem only when a person is experiencing a lot of false alarms—a situation that is common for people who struggle with excessive anxiety.

The amygdala (an almond-shaped mass of neurons that play a key role in processing emotion, fear in particular) can become hypersensitive to feelings of anxiety. This tends to happen in situations of severe trauma or chronic stress. "Cortisol [a hormone that is released when we're under stress] and glutamate [a neurotransmitter that carries messages in the brain] act to excite the amygdala, and the more it is excited, the more easily it is triggered," explains John Arden, author of *Rewire Your Brain: Think Your Way to a Better Life*.

But just as our brains can learn to become too sensitive to feelings of anxiety, they can learn to become less sensitive too. This is because we quite literally have the power to change our own brains, through our thoughts and actions. As Linda Graham

> It has helped a lot to gently steer her toward independence in all areas of life, because it shows she's a competent kid who can handle whatever comes her way. At the same time, it's crucial that, when she's feeling overwhelmed by a particular task, I stop and deal with those feelings and then help her by breaking the task down into small steps for her. She wants me to do everything with her, so I'm careful to offer ongoing support and continual check-ins while still insisting she work on her own in between.
>
> **Alison, mother of Charlotte, who has been diagnosed with an anxiety disorder**

explains in her book *Bouncing Back: Rewiring Your Brain for Maximum Resilience and Well-Being*, "Because of neuroplasticity [the brain's ability to change itself], we can always create new pathways and circuits that are more resilient and effective in responding to the challenges in our lives." A child who is struggling with anxiety doesn't have to struggle with anxiety forever. He can learn how to train his brain to be less reactive and more resilient.

So, what can you do to help your child manage feelings of anxiety? Try the following suggestions, for starters.

> As a single footstep will not make a path on the earth, so a single thought will not make a pathway in the mind. To make a deep physical path, we walk again and again. To make a deep mental path, we must think over and over the kind of thoughts we wish to dominate our lives.
> **Henry David Thoreau**

### Teach Your Child How to Recognize the Physical Sensations of Anxiety

When she is becoming anxious, she may notice that her heart is beating faster, she's breathing more rapidly, she has butterflies in her stomach, her hands and feet feel cold, her mouth is dry, and she feels restless. Sometimes symptoms of illness can be mistaken for feelings of anxiety. Ditto for feelings of happy excitement. Take note of your child's physical complaints, like headaches and stomachaches. Remind your child that these symptoms could be her body trying to tell her something. Maybe she's worried about school or a falling out with a friend?

### Teach Your Child about Anxiety and How It Affects Our Bodies and Our Brains

First, anxiety affects our thought processes. Anxious feelings can cloud our thinking, skew our thinking to negative, and encourage us to engage in avoidant behavior—which sounds like a good strategy for reducing anxiety until you stop to consider that problems, and worries, tend to grow when they're left to languish in the dark. The key to taming your amygdala—to rewiring your brain to be less anxious and more resilient—is to gradually teach yourself to cope with situations that made you anxious in the past. As Arden puts it: "Avoiding avoidance and maximizing exposure reduces anxiety in the long run." This does not mean, however, that you should buy your arachnophobic child a giant pet spider in an effort to help him deal with his fears. Exposure therapy is best left to the professionals. Instead, encourage him to challenge some of the thinking that may be causing that phobia about spiders to keep getting bigger and bigger. Ask questions like "What is the worst thing that could happen if a spider were to crawl on you?" "If this were to happen, what could you do to deal with the situation?"

Second, the bodily sensations that are triggered by feelings of anxiety may be uncomfortable (dry mouth, a racing heart), but they are rarely harmful. So your child doesn't have to feel anxious about anxious feelings causing her harm. (Hey, that's one less thing to feel anxious about.)

> Our son has tremendous anxiety and worries about things all the time. I waver between wanting to be so prepared and organized that nothing can go wrong and thinking it's better for him to learn how to cope with life's unexpected curveballs. It's a daily struggle.
>
> **Laura, whose son, Gabriel, has been diagnosed with Asperger syndrome and is currently being assessed for OCD**

Third, it takes time for the body to return to a state of calm after it's been jacked up on anxious emotions. You can't just flip a switch and turn off feelings of anxiety when you're finished with them. There's a recovery period involved.

Understanding how anxiety works at a physiological level will help your child learn how to take action to calm herself when she feels her anxiety levels ramping up, like going for a run around the block or engaging in a favorite hobby. Here are some strategies you can help her learn to use.

## Teach Your Child to Name the Emotion

Labeling a panicky feeling as anxiety helps to tame the emotion. This is because labeling an emotion activates the thinking part of your brain (the left prefrontal cortex), calming the part of your brain that specializes in emotions like fear (the amygdala).

## Help Your Child Deal with the Problem

Doing something constructive to deal with the problem will reassure the amygdala that it's done its job—you're paying attention to the perceived threat—and now it can go chill out. For a child who is freaking out about the big project he has due for school, it could be a matter of breaking that project into smaller pieces (coming up with a list of questions to research, creating an outline, writing a first draft, and then editing the final report). For an adolescent who is feeling anxious about having a difficult conversation with a teacher, it could be a matter of role playing that conversation with a friend or parent first.

## Help Your Child Practice Worry Triage

Focusing on how anxious and worried you feel or indulging in worst-case scenario thinking (sometimes called catastrophizing) doesn't make things better. It makes things worse. A helpful way to break out of this all-too-common rut is to subject your worries to what Michael A. Southam-Gerow, author of *Emotion Regulation in Children and Adolescents: A Practitioner's Guide*, calls "worry triage." He suggests asking yourself a series of questions designed to determine whether you can take action on a particular worry right now, whether you can take action at some point but not right now, or whether you probably don't have any control over these worries at all. For example, your child might ask herself:

- "How much control do I have over this situation?"
- "What steps can I take to solve this problem?"
- "What will happen if I stop thinking about this situation?"
- "What will happen if I do nothing about this situation?"
- "How much less likely is that to occur if I worry about it?"
- "How important is this problem, as compared to other items on my worry list?"

Other techniques that can be helpful in starting a conversation about worries include:

- Drawing a stress-o-meter—a thermometer with gradations from 0 to 100%—and asking your child to mark on the thermometer just how worried she is right now, so that the two of you can talk about what's behind those worries.
- Creating a worry tree—your child can record his worries on paper leaves and then hang those worries on the tree so that he doesn't have to carry them around in his head.

## Call Off the Fight-or-Flight Response

Deep breathing, the kind that engages the diaphragm so that you feel your stomach expand, can help to relax you, calming the fight-or-flight response that is triggered by high levels of anxiety. Talk to your child about the difference between "full belly breathing" (the relaxing kind, which gives you a rounded belly) and "Superman breathing" (the stressed kind, which gives you a puffed out, superhero-like chest). Encourage your child to practice other types of relaxation techniques (see Chapter 5).

### Take a Break from Your Worries

While avoidance is one of the worst ways of dealing with anxiety, there's nothing wrong with taking a temporary break from your worries, particularly if you do so in a way that makes it clear to your worries that you're not trying to hide from them or run away for good. Do something fun so that the worries fly out of your head. And if they happen to fly back, don't panic. Acknowledge their presence and get on with the business of having fun.

Imagine yourself taking off a backpack full of worries and leaving it by the front door until morning or mentally downloading the worries from inside your head onto your computer drive so your computer (the high-tech equivalent of a Guatemalan worry doll) can handle your worries for you while you take a break.

Treat anxiety as something outside the child, like an imaginary monster, suggests Walter Mittelstaedt, adjunct clinical faculty at the University of Waterloo in Ontario, Canada, and director of the university's Centre for Mental Health Research. He recommends that parents and kids work together in this way so they can team up to chase worry away.

### Recognize That Your Child Might Need Additional Help

While there's plenty you can do to help your child deal with her anxiety, it's important to recognize when your child might benefit from some outside assistance as well. A trained professional in children's mental health can help a child cope with anxious feelings while acquiring greater courage and confidence. Techniques include recalling situations in which the child acted bravely or sharing stories about the brave acts of other people (especially family members and friends). And you might get help in teaching your child to develop his attention regulation skills. Children who are able to take breaks from the source of their anxiety by shifting their focus to other activities tend to be better at managing their anxiety. Another technique that you might find help with is gradually exposing your child to situations that provoke feelings of anxiety, so that she can learn to overcome such feelings over time.

> We had a lot of strategies for the anxiety, like having a card laminated with a list of things she could ask herself before deciding something was beyond doing herself and having a bingo card with a lot of different ways of self-managing when anxiety hit, since she couldn't remember those strategies in the middle of it.
>
> **Heather, mother of four children with various challenges, including Fiona, who struggles with anxiety**

## Developing the Skills
## That Make Change Possible

Your child isn't acting the way he does because he wants to be difficult. He's acting the way he does because he believes it's the only option he has right now.

Most children who struggle to manage intense emotions do so because they have underdeveloped skills in one or more of the following areas: language-processing skills, emotion-processing skills, cognitive flexibility skills, social skills, and executive skills (the higher-order thinking skills that control activities like organizing and planning). "Executive functioning can be compared to a command or control center in our brains that oversees actions and mental operations, notes Leah M. Kuypers in *The Zones of Regulation: A Curriculum Designed to Foster Self-Regulation and Emotional Control*. "Numerous mental operations fall under executive functioning, but some that are influential to the ability to self-regulate are attention shifting (attending to two or more activities simultaneously . . .), working memory (updating and purging 'files' in the brain with new information), internalization of speech (self-talk), flexible thinking (considering multiple options), planning (organizing actions and executing a plan in order to reach desired goals), and inhibition (impulse control)."

Coming to this realization—that your child's behavior is the result of a skills deficit as opposed to a deliberate decision to act up—can be a total game changer for you and your child. It means you can let go of any feelings of guilt, resentment, or blame that you may have been carrying (and, frankly, those feelings become pretty burdensome pretty quickly). Instead, you can start feeling compassionate toward yourself and your child (you're each doing the best you can in a tough situation) while simultaneously switching into problem-solving mode. As Ross W. Greene and J. Stuart Ablon note in their groundbreaking book *Treating Explosive Kids: The Collaborative Problem-Solving Approach*, "Identifying the specific lagging skills underlying a child's explosive and noncompliant behavior accomplishes two crucial missions. First, adults are

> I get frustrated when my husband gets angry about something Laura can't control. I get frustrated with myself when I get angry at Laura about something she can't control, or a new fixation pops up that is particularly trying. She can't help it, so I have to find a way to cope, even when she's singing Hannah Montana songs off-key over and over and over and over.
>
> **Lisa, mother of Laura, who is currently awaiting diagnosis**

# What Every Parent Needs to Know about Executive Skills

| Type of cognitive skill | Behavioral symptoms when there is a deficit in this area | How to help your child manage this deficit |
|---|---|---|
| **Executive skills (general):** high-level brain functions that look after organization, planning, and shifting from one way of thinking to another | • Difficulty managing transitions between activities<br>• Difficulty organizing thoughts<br>• Difficulty following the steps in a multistep task | • Provide advance warning of upcoming transitions between activities.<br>• Teach your child how to chunk ideas (break them into smaller, more manageable pieces) and stay on track with deadlines at school—or hire a homework coach to spend a couple of hours a week working with him on these tasks.<br>• Create lists or pictographs to help your child follow the steps in a process. |
| **Response inhibition:** the ability to inhibit a response (e.g., stopping yourself from blurting out answers or hitting other people), a specific type of executive skill | • Difficulty waiting for it to be one's turn<br>• Difficulty self-censoring insensitive or inappropriate comments | • Give your child opportunities to practice waiting her turn in a safe, supportive environment.<br>• Play games like Pop-up Pirate, which features unexpected twists, so your child can practice dealing with the unexpected.<br>• Help your child understand how her comments affect other people and what she could do to prevent herself from blurting out similar comments in the future (e.g., distracting herself). |
| **Working memory capacity:** having a workspace in your brain that allows you to think through ideas before acting on them, a specific type of executive skill that is thought to affect the functioning of most other executive skills | • Difficulty keeping track of belongings<br>• Difficulty remembering rules<br>• Difficulty following all or part of verbal instructions<br>• Difficulty thinking through an emotional response before responding | • Provide your child with tools that will allow him to keep track of important information (calendars, checklists, notebooks) and teach him to choose cues in his environment that can help him retrieve the important information he needs at various times (e.g., by placing his morning checklist on the refrigerator door so he sees it and remembers to review it).<br>• Encourage your child to do one thing at a time, as opposed to multitasking, which increases the demand on working memory.<br>• Encourage your child to develop his working memory skills by scanning a page in a magazine and circling as |

many instances of the word *the* as he can spot in 30 seconds; by trying to find Waldo in a *Where's Waldo?* book, or by listing six of his favorite songs out loud and then repeating them back to you in reverse order.

| | | |
|---|---|---|
| **Language-processing skills:** being able to process language efficiently and effectively in the brain | • Difficulty expressing thoughts, needs, or concerns in words<br>• Difficulty understanding what others have said<br>• Difficulty responding to questions promptly<br>• Difficulty defining or expressing emotions | • Establish eye contact with your child before you begin speaking.<br>• Break information into "chunks" (e.g., one chunk for each step in a task).<br>• Repeat instructions or have your child summarize instructions for you.<br>• Encourage your child to ask for clarification whenever necessary.<br>• Allow extra time for your child to process and recall information.<br>• Make emotion a topic of conversation in your home (see the "What You Can Do" section of this chapter). |
| **Emotional regulation skills:** being able to monitor and control emotions so that emotions meet the needs of a particular situation | • Difficulty remaining calm when frustrated<br>• Difficulty maintaining a positive or neutral mood (may be cranky, grouchy, irritable; anxious, nervous, and worried; or sad, tired, and lacking in energy)<br>• Difficulty recovering from disappointments | • Identify situations that trigger emotions in your child and help her prepare for such situations by developing a script of things she can say to herself ("If I get stuck, I can ask for help.").<br>• Use a rating scale to rate the intensity of emotions (see page 121).<br>• Use puppets to act out a variety of situations and emotions and encourage your child to experiment with possible solutions to the problems.<br>• Play games like Cross the Line (where the child walks across the room, acting out one emotion until he crosses a real or imaginary line, at which point he starts acting out a different emotion). This game helps children understand that their entire bodies are involved in relaying emotions.<br>• Modify the environment to reduce the number of problem situations your child encounters.<br>• Teach your child stress management and coping strategies (see Chapter 5). |

| Type of cognitive skill | Behavioral symptoms when there is a deficit in this area | How to help your child manage this deficit |
| --- | --- | --- |
| **Cognitive flexibility skills:** being a flexible thinker as opposed to a very rules-based thinker | • Difficulty considering changes to routines, plans, ideas, or rules<br>• Difficulty appreciating other people's points of view<br>• Difficulty dealing with situations that are unpredictable, uncertain, or ambiguous<br>• Difficulty considering a variety of solutions to a problem | • Provide advance warning of changes that you know about. Help your child develop scripts that she can play in her head if she encounters an unplanned—and unwelcome—change (e.g., "I can handle this").<br>• Provide step-by-step support or guidance as your child works his way through an unfamiliar task.<br>• Help your child see the good things about having more than one person's perspective on things, having something unexpected happen, and considering more than one solution to a problem. Encourage your child to experiment with these concepts. |
| **Social skills:** understanding the unwritten rules of social behavior; exhibiting empathy | • Difficulty noticing or reading social cues<br>• Difficulty with basic social skills (how to start a conversation, how to seek attention in an appropriate way)<br>• Difficulty understanding how one's behavior is affecting others<br>• Difficulty with empathy | • Identify your child's social skills deficits.<br>• Choose a single behavior to focus on changing initially, as opposed to trying to target a range of behaviors all at the same time.<br>• Explain to your child what he needs to know about this particular behavior (how to start or join a conversation; how to seek attention without annoying other people).<br>• Give your child a chance to learn more about social skills through role playing social scenarios and by discussing social situations (those drawn both from real life and from books and movies).<br>• Provide your child with constructive feedback about how his behavior affects other people.<br>• Model and encourage empathy.<br>• Give your child a chance to participate in individual or group activities that don't rely on the ability to read social cues (running, swimming, skiing, art, drama). |

*Sources*: Data from Ross W. Greene and J. Stuart Ablon, *Treating Explosive Kids: The Collaborative Problem-Solving Approach* (New York: Guilford Press, 2006); Peg Dawson and Richard Guare, *Executive Skills in Children and Adolescents, Second Edition: A Practical Guide to Assessment and Intervention* (New York: Guilford Press, 2010).

helped to understand that the child's difficulties are not due to a deficit in motivation or to adult ineptitude but rather to a deficit in cognitive skills, and therefore programs based on rewarding and punishing are unlikely to achieve satisfactory results because incentive-based programs do not train lacking cognitive skills. Second, adults are pointed directly to the specific cognitive skills that do need to be trained."

So, how can you tell which types of cognitive skills your child may lack, and what can you do to address any deficits, to reduce the amount of frustration your child and you have been experiencing? By finding out more about each of these specific cognitive deficits.

The chart on pages 130–132 summarizes the key symptoms associated with some of the key cognitive deficits that are associated with mental, emotional, and behavioral problems in children. You may have observed some of these symptoms in your child, or a psychoeducational assessment may have identified (or will in future identify) one or more of these deficits. When you're considering the various strategies listed in the third column, be sure to zero in on the ones that are most suited to your child's developmental stage and abilities.

Once you know what you're dealing with, you can begin to work on addressing the underlying issues by modifying your child's environment, helping your child learn ways to compensate for his deficits (see Peg Dawson and Richard Guare's *Smart but Scattered* series of books), and giving him opportunities to work on strengthening his skills—with some behind-the-scenes support from you. (See the chart on pages 130–132 for specific tips.) Remind yourself that children, like adults, need the opportunity to act independently and learn from their mistakes in order to acquire new skills. Rome wasn't built in a day—and your child won't magically acquire a new set of skills overnight.

## You Have the Power

Once again, when it comes to guiding your child through the emotional storms, your approach to parenting is key. You want your child to know that you are on his side, that you understand why he has been acting the way he has been acting (his behavior makes sense, given the frustration he has been facing), and that you're committed to doing everything you can to make things better for him, starting right now.

Validating his feelings and responding with compassion for the struggle he has been experiencing will take your relationship to a new level while opening up new possibilities for health and healing. As Haim G. Ginott wrote in his classic book *Teacher and Child: A Book for Parents and Teachers* nearly 40 years ago, "I have come to the frightening conclusion that I am the decisive element. It is my personal approach that creates the climate. It is my daily mood that makes the weather. I possess tremendous power to make life miserable or joyous. I can be a tool of torture or an instrument of inspiration, I can humiliate or humor, hurt or heal."

Yes, you have that power.

# Part III

# Your Family

When your child is struggling with a mental health challenge, you can feel like the rest of your life is out of whack. Your relationships with your partner and your other children may suffer. Your health may deteriorate. You may feel as if your entire life is falling apart. It is easy to allow the needs of the child who is struggling to zap every ounce of your physical and emotional reserves, leaving you with little left for yourself, let alone anyone else.

Fortunately, it doesn't have to be this way.

You can take action to nurture your relationships with your partner and your other children. You can commit to making your health a priority as well—a decision that will reap dividends for other family members at the same time.

Consider the next two chapters a call to action on the relationship and health fronts—a reminder of the importance of nurturing your relationships with other family members and safeguarding your own health.

In Chapter 8, we'll talk about how your other children and your partner may be faring and what you can do to ensure that your family is strengthened rather than destroyed by the challenges you are facing right now.

Then, in Chapter 9, we'll look at how leading a healthy lifestyle (ensuring that you're getting enough sleep, making room in your life for physical activity and fun, and eating well) can maximize health.

The strategies outlined in this chapter are designed to improve the health of all family members, including the health of the child who is struggling.

It makes perfect sense that your child's struggles are front and center in your life right now. *How could they not be?* But, that said, you don't want your child's struggles to eclipse your relationships with other people or to compromise your own health. It's possible to take good care of the child who is struggling and to take good care of yourself and other family members too.

I hope you'll be inspired by the advice offered by other families who have walked this path and that you'll walk away with fresh ideas for sustaining your health and relationships as you continue to weather the storm.

# 8

# Family Matters

Mental health challenges don't affect just the child who is struggling. They affect other family members too. And the only way to weather this storm as a family is to ensure that all family members receive the love and support they need. The best way to make that happen is by thinking about your child's challenges as a challenge for the entire family, says Andrew, whose son David has been diagnosed with schizophrenia: "Try not to think of it as your child as having 'the problem.' Your *family* has the problem—the problem of having to live well with a vulnerable family member."

> Mental illness is a family struggle. It affects everyone in the family.
> —Susan, mother of Jacob, who struggles with anxiety

## Taking Care of Your Other Children

It's tough enough to try to make sense of a family member's mental illness when you're an adult. It's tougher still when you're a kid and the family member in question is your brother or sister. Add to that the fact that family rules and routines may change overnight to accommodate your sibling's needs, your sibling may end up with special rules that don't seem fair or reasonable to you, and you may be worried about what the future holds for your brother or sister and it's easy to see why siblings of children who are struggling often end up feeling stressed and frustrated themselves.

Christine, whose son, Will, has been diagnosed with severe ADHD and an anxiety disorder, remembers feeling bad about the way things at home affected her daughter when her son's struggles were at their worst. "We stopped inviting the children's friends over," she recalls. "We never knew what kind of day Will would have, so I didn't feel we could really have people over, in case he threw a fit. We stopped planning daylong outings, again in case Will had a very bad day and we had to come home right away. . . . When things were at their worst, I felt completely hopeless. I was afraid that we would become even more isolated. I was also sad for my daughter, who has no social, behavioral, or mental health issues, yet was becoming more isolated as a result of her brother's mental illness."

Sometimes feelings of resentment can arise between siblings.

"Our oldest felt like Braeden got all of our time and energy. He felt neglected," recalls Stephanie, whose son has been diagnosed with OCD and ADHD.

"My other children love their brother, but at times they have been so frustrated and angry with him. They didn't know how to deal with him," says Claire, whose son Owen has been diagnosed with bipolar disorder, a personality disorder, and extreme anxiety.

Even if the siblings seem to be coping, it's hard not to worry about how they may be affected over the long term. "My most significant regret is that I probably wasn't there enough for my other two kids," says Darlene, whose daughter Alicia was hospitalized for extended periods of time for treatment of her eating disorder. "Andrea—at the ripe old age of 9—ended up being asked to take care of her 8-year-old brother. They're the ones I think are left with the lasting scars from this experience."

How can parents support their other children in dealing with the fallout from a sibling's challenges?

### Recognize That Children May React in a Variety of Ways

When a sibling develops or is diagnosed with a psychiatric disorder, it's bound to be disruptive for the other children in the family. Some may be confused or upset by the changes in their sibling's behavior—and possibly even traumatized by episodes of extreme behavior. Others may resent all the attention that is being directed toward their sibling. Some may be afraid of developing a similar disorder themselves. Others may attempt to become "the perfect child" so that they won't contribute any more stress to the family. How a particular child reacts will be determined, in part, by his age at the onset of his sibling's challenges, his relationship with that sibling prior to that time, and how other family members respond. A very young child may pick up on the fact that something is wrong, even if he doesn't know exactly what that is, and he may respond with heightened emotions and behaviors, such as being extra clingy, extra cranky, extra active, or withdrawn. A teenager, on the other hand, might have a better understanding of the challenges involved but might be trying to mask feelings of anxiety or anger or resentment, leading to a tendency to withdraw from the family or seek the attention of parents by acting out in unexpected and inappropriate ways.

### Accept Whatever It Is Your Other Children Are Feeling toward Their Sibling Who Is Struggling

Don't criticize or shame a child if she is feeling angry or resentful. These feelings are common and make sense. Instead, listen with kindness, suspend judgment (see Chapter 6 for more on nonjudgmental parenting), and focus on helping that child develop coping skills, including strategies for coping with disruptive behaviors from a sibling, dealing with rude or intrusive questions from other people, and managing her own feelings.

### Help Your Child Understand That the Needs of Individual Family Members Shift over Time

Remind your child that when he was a baby, he needed, and received, round-the-clock care from you because he wasn't able to take care of himself. A person with a broken leg may need a little extra help temporarily. Everyone needs different kinds of help at different times. The good thing about being part of a family is that people are able to pitch in and help you when you need it most, and you're able to return the favor in their time of need. You can also reassure your child that you'll do your best to be there for him the next time he needs a little extra love and attention and then honor that promise by finding ways to spend one-on-one time with each of your children on a regular basis, so that they may continue to feel your love and caring.

### Ensure That Your Other Children Have Access to Support

"Get family counseling," suggests Stephanie, mother of Braeden. "Counseling can help siblings understand, and it can keep parents from babying or giving too much time to the child with the diagnosis." It can also provide a neutral forum for setting ground rules for issues like teasing. "We've had to impress upon David's closest sibling, his brother and best friend William, that picking on him for his attention issues was not okay," says Marie, whose son David has been diagnosed with a severe combined form of ADHD, sensory integration disorder, and two learning disabilities.

### *Don't Overlook the Positive Side*

Growing up with a sibling with a mental health problem can lead children to become more tolerant, more compassionate, and more mature than others who have not been faced with the same challenge early in life. Laura, whose son, Gabriel, has been diagnosed with Asperger syndrome (which became part of the umbrella term *autism spectrum disorder* as of DSM-5) and is currently being assessed for OCD, has watched this play out in her own family. "Gabriel's sisters are younger than him," she explains. "He is very nice to them—probably much more so than a 'typical' brother would be, so they've actually benefited from Gabriel's Asperger's. My older daughter does seem to feel a strong sense of responsibility for her brother. She is only 20 months younger than him and has taken on a caretaker role with him. She will often patiently explain a social nuance to him or reassure him when he's feeling particularly anxious. It's lovely to see. As a mother, I'm happy to know that she will look out for him in life."

## Staying Connected as a Couple

Disagreements about how to handle parenting issues can cause friction in a couple relationship at the best of times, and dealing with the fallout of a child's mental health challenges can hardly be described as the best of times. Of course, this assumes that you're in a couple relationship right now or that, if estranged from your child's other parent, you're still actively coparenting. If that is not the case—you're a single parent and/or your child's other parent is no longer involved in the child's life—you'll want to tap into support from extended family members and/or create your own circle of support by surrounding yourself with helpful and caring friends. See Chapter 12 for more about getting support at home, at work, and in the community, as well as the related discussions elsewhere in this chapter.

But assuming you *are* part of a couple relationship, you'll want to work at staying connected with your partner as the two of you face your child's challenges together.

That isn't always easy.

"My husband and son have struggled in their relationship over the years, and the new OCD issues haven't helped," says Laura, mother of Gabriel. "Although my husband understands 'on paper' that Gabriel isn't choosing these behaviors, he seems to lose patience with him much more quickly than I do."

"It's been challenging," adds Lisa, whose daughter, Laura, is in the process of being diagnosed but who exhibits many symptoms of OCD and anxiety. "I'm the researcher, the reader, the advocate. Mental illness doesn't scare me. My husband was raised in a 'my way or the highway' house, and he reverts to that, sometimes about things our daughter can't help because of her challenges. He gets mad at me when I get better results [with her], but I've been doing the reading and the talking and the research and the reaching out. He doesn't want to do it, doesn't want to listen to me, and then gets mad when I get results."

"The diagnosis caused a significant amount of tension in my marriage," notes Leigh, whose son, Skyler, has been diagnosed with ADHD, anxiety, and depression. "My husband did not always agree with my advocacy and felt that some of this was just bad behavior: that discipline would be the solution. He was also not always home because of his work schedule and had the expectation that I would provide discipline follow-through that I didn't always believe in. I felt that I knew my son best because I was the one who spent the most time with him."

"It's affected my married life," adds Meg, whose son, Jayden, has been diagnosed with an anxiety disorder. "We are both so tired all the time. We try to get time together, but this often takes up a lot of space in our relationship."

The situation may be frustrating, but it isn't hopeless, says Will's mother, Christine. "If you and your partner have the same views on mental illness and treatment, you will remain connected. I was very fortunate in this regard. My husband and I worked together as a team. We always remained close."

So how do some couples manage to stay connected, despite extraordinarily challenging circumstances?

## Work Together and Make Time for Fun

Andrew, father of David, offers some tips on staying connected as a couple while you're dealing with the ongoing stress of a child's mental health challenges. "Seek out positive connection on a regular basis," he advises. "Make time for fun and the various relationships in the family. Couples in particular should try to find time to talk, have fun, and work out issues as they come up. Try to aim for teamwork and mostly being on the same page, although disagreements are inevitable and, in fact, can deepen the conversation and lead to good decisions. Practice forgiveness and realize that some 'bad behavior' on the part of the other is about the stress and baggage that come from being under pressure at times. Keep family rituals and traditions or create some new ones. Stay close to nature. Enjoy good food and, maybe above all else, laugh and look for the funny stuff in even the darkest times."

### Find Time for Each Other and Practice Kindness

Don't expect a relationship to stay on track on its own. You have to work at staying connected, notes Andrea, whose youngest son, Jack, has been diagnosed with Tourette syndrome, bipolar disorder, OCD, and a learning disability. "My husband and I always made sure we had a date night every Friday night. My advice? Schedule it and book it so you know you have that time to look forward to. By the time that evening rolls around, you're going to need it. And be kind to each other. You're both going through so much and you each deal with the grief and sadness differently."

Cheyenne, whose daughter, Keisha, has been diagnosed with ADHD and anxiety, agrees that erring on the side of kindness in your treatment of your partner is key: "I've come to accept what he can and can't do and to stop blaming him for what he can't. It's not bad, it's not wrong, it's not his fault, it doesn't mean he's a bad dad. It's simply that different people can handle different things."

### Consider Couple Therapy

If you find you're running into conflict in your relationship, you may want to consider going for couple therapy. A therapist can provide a safe haven for you and your partner to discuss sensitive and emotionally volatile issues. You might need some guidance to sort out the different roles you're taking in supporting your child (perhaps one of you is playing a more active role in advocating for your child than the other as a result of schedules or personalities). Or maybe you find yourselves disagreeing about your approach to parenting a child who is struggling. Taking these issues to a counselor together for an objective viewpoint can really help.

> My son's health and behavior affected our home life and my marriage. I was married to his stepdad when he was 2 years old. They had a great relationship until he was 15. His stepdad could not understand or deal with William's behavior or my depression either. He tried to kick him out of the house at 16 for breaking curfew. He came back until he was 18 but moved out then. I don't think he would have moved out so young were he not depressed or if his stepdad were more supportive."
>
> —Joanne, whose son William has been diagnosed with depression

### Focus on Coparenting

It's important to work on maintaining a peaceful and functional coparenting relationship with your child's other parent, even if the two of you are no longer part of a couple relationship. If counseling or therapy is not an option, be sure to communicate regularly and make a point of keeping your communications focused on the shared goal of helping your child. This will help to ensure that the dialogue remains positive and constructive.

## Creating a Circle of Support

Your group of friends may undergo a bit of a shuffle in the aftermath of your child's diagnosis. You may find that some people distance themselves because they simply don't know how to react or what to say.

"I think our social circle got reorganized somewhat as people who were uneasy with our situation backed away, but close friends and family showed a willingness to get more involved—and that was essential and appreciated," recalls Andrew, father of David.

"As soon as there was any diagnosis—a label—people ran," says Mark, whose son, Dawson, has been diagnosed with reactive attachment disorder, an anxiety disorder, and a moderate developmental disability. "We had a large circle of friends—some with children, some without—and we could see the cloud of smoke behind them as they ran out the door. . . . It makes me sad that some of our friends will never see what a remarkable young man our son is growing up to be."

Some parents find themselves pulling away from other people out of fear of being judged—particularly if their child's behavior has become extreme: "I was so embarrassed and I didn't know what to do," recalls Carolyn, whose son Ezra has been diagnosed with pervasive developmental delay, ADHD, anxiety, and depression and has had conflicts with the law resulting from his social skills deficits. "I'm a good mom, and by definition the kids of good moms aren't arrested. It's not something you bring up at the mommy circle."

Rebecca can relate to those feelings. "I've pulled away from a lot of friends who have neurotypical kids or who just don't get it," says Rebecca. "I've also pulled away from my parents because they think I am overreacting or that Madalyn is just going through a stage."

One of the biggest challenges that Sandra has faced in parenting her daughter Sophie (who has been diagnosed with moderate autism with global developmental delays) has been "never feeling like anyone else understands how difficult it is, and [their thinking] that it's your poor parenting that makes it worse," she says. "I don't give in to my child to make our lives difficult. I do it because I know what to give in to and what to stand up to in order to make our lives easier."

Claire, mother of Owen, can relate to that feeling: "We have been so surprised at how people have judged us, and who. Honestly, we are not too trusting."

It's particularly difficult when the people passing the judgment are family members whose unconditional love and support you crave, notes Tami, whose son Adam has been diagnosed with ADHD. "We have a hard time going out as a family to do any kind of planned activity, as Adam will not have the patience for it. Holiday dinners are particularly tough. He gets bored, acts out, and, of course, he's coming off his meds in the evening. This has created some friction with extended family, who (I think) have a hard time understanding that this is not simply a discipline issue."

Sandra, Sophie's mother, offers this advice to friends and family members who might be tempted to offer unsolicited advice to parents who have a child who is struggling with a mental illness: "Be supportive without offering unsolicited advice. If you haven't been there, no amount of books or things you've seen on the Internet are going to make you completely understand what I'm going through. Please stop telling me how you would do it better. I'm doing my best. You want to help? Ask me what I need and then give me that, not something else you think I need instead. Don't add to my stress by putting more demands on me."

### Help Others Help You

Helping friends and family members figure out what they can do to help is definitely worth the effort, notes Andrea. "Really think about what kind of help you would benefit from and let people know what you need. People often feel bad about what you are experiencing but don't know what to do to help." Try to be as specific as possible when spelling out your needs. Let them know what would help most, whether it be taking your struggling child's sibling to see a movie, helping you catch up on yard work and other to-do list chores, coming with you to an important meeting at your child's school and taking notes, or simply encouraging you to relax and take the best possible care of yourself. This kind of hands-on help and moral support is particularly important if you're parenting on your own.

Of course, some friends and neighbors find it difficult to step forward and offer this kind of practical support when a family is dealing with a mental health crisis as opposed to a different type of health crisis—which is why combating stigma is key to allowing families to tap into much-needed support.

"Mental illness is not a casserole illness," explains Liza Long, author of *The Price of Silence* and mother of a teenager who has been diagnosed with bipolar disorder. And if we're going to make it a casserole illness—the kind of illness where neighbors drop off casseroles to show their support for families who are struggling—we need to normalize our reactions to mental illness.

Andrew Solomon, author of *The Noonday Demon: An Atlas of Depression* and *Far from the Tree: Parents, Children, and the Search for Identity*, agrees: "These conditions are not contagious, and they shouldn't frighten people as much as they do—and, more significantly, they don't reflect anybody's moral weakness or shortcoming. They are, in fact, conditions that occur frequently, that respond to treatment, and that are organic illnesses of the brain. There's no reason for the people who are reporting them to feel embarrassed, and there's no reason for the casserole-producing neighbors to feel like the whole thing is so shameful and uncomfortable that they can't respond."

## *Help Others Understand—and Understand Their Limitations*

While you're asking for help, look for opportunities to educate friends and family members about your child's challenges and your family's struggles. Think of how much knowledge and insight you have acquired as a result of this experience and then pass along some of that hard-earned wisdom to others who care about you.

Just don't expect miracles from yourself or others. Even when friends and family members *are* being supportive, simple logistics or time pressures can make it difficult to maintain relationships when a child is having a difficult time.

"I cannot leave Fiona alone for long periods of time," explains Mary, whose daughter has been diagnosed with bipolar disorder. "Once I went to a business dinner and she had an anxiety attack. When I turned my phone on 2 hours later, I had 100 missed calls. I have to weigh social invitations carefully and often only accept if I can bring her with me, which is not particularly relaxing for me."

"You may have to put some [relationships] on hold," says Christine, mother of Will. "My good friends understood when I disappeared for the better part of a year. They knew my family was going through something difficult, even though they didn't know what it was. And they were there for me when things got better and I was ready to reconnect. You just have to do the best you can for yourself. That might mean missing more than a few birthday and holiday celebrations because you're just not feeling up to it. Be honest with the people you care about. Tell them things at home are hard right now and you need to focus on that for a while. Your good friends will understand."

Those are the friendships that are to be treasured, because they will form your circle of support as you weather the storm.

"You quickly learn who your true friends are," says Claire, mother of Owen. "True friends love you and will listen, even when they have heard it many times, even when you have dealt with your child's illness for a long time. They will not judge you, and they will always care enough to ask how you and your child are doing."

"Anyone who was supportive was golden to me," adds Tami, Adam's mother. "Friends who would listen and not judge. My mother, who had gone through so many of the same experiences with my brother when he was growing up, has been my rock."

"I have a coworker I have worked with for over 20 years," says Mary, mother of Fiona, who has been diagnosed with bipolar disorder, and Janine, who has a mild intellectual disability and is on the autism spectrum. "If I call and need someone to come to the emergency department with me to help out, she will come. She is the person I unload on when things become too much. She understands what I am going through. I find that my own moods reflect Fiona's ups and downs and that there is sometimes a risk that my own health will deteriorate with hers. I need someone to lean on and remind me that I am not my daughter's illness and that tomorrow is another day."

"We have generally invested in those relationships that are obviously supportive over time and pulled back from ones where there are signs of ambivalence or outright disconnection," says David's father, Andrew. "Why waste time? Life is too short to waste time feeling bad that not everyone is willing or able to be there for you in a way that makes a difference. We have been blessed with a lot of support, so we are not desperate to seek it from just anyone."

"The blessing in this is that you're going to make new, wonderful friends that you never would have made otherwise," says Cheyenne, whose daughter, Keisha, has been diagnosed with ADHD and anxiety. "The only people that really understand are people who have been through it. Anyone with a kid with challenges can relate and is going to be supportive."

For more on what's involved in forging these life-sustaining bonds, see Chapter 12.

## No Family Is Perfect

You'll find it easier to reach out for support from others—and to help your child create a much-needed circle of support (a topic we'll be returning to in Chapter 12)—if you remind yourself that every family has its struggles. The myth of the perfect family is just that: a myth. "We seem to have this idea in our heads about how a family should look or how others should behave," says Tami, mother of Adam. "I think it's only gotten worse with social media, where people post all the lovely photos of their smiling families enjoying all kinds of holidays and activities. But obviously people only post the happy stuff. They're not going to start snapping photos when their kid is mid-meltdown or when their kid is called to the principal's office."

Don't make the mistake of assuming that your family is different or defective simply because your child is struggling. That kind of thinking causes you to feel disconnected from the rest of the world and makes it more difficult for you to reach out for the very types of support your family needs right now. "Our fears and self-judgments are like blinders that often prevent us from seeing the hands that are being held out to help us," writes Kristin Neff in *Self-Compassion: Stop Beating Yourself Up and Leave Insecurity Behind*. "When our troubled, painful experiences are framed by the recognition that countless others have undergone similar hardships, the blow is softened. The pain still hurts, but it doesn't become compounded by feelings of separation."

# 9

# Lifestyle Matters

It almost seems too good to be true: the idea that taking better care of our physical health could have a far-reaching impact on our mental health. And yet, when you think about it, it makes all the sense in the world. When we give our bodies what they actually need—adequate sleep, regular physical activity, time for fun and relaxation, top-quality fuel in the form of good nutrition—why wouldn't they reward us by functioning at their best, both mentally and physically?

> Diet and lifestyle are much more important than I thought in helping someone with a mental illness.
>
> —Sari, mother of Ryan, who has been diagnosed with ADHD, and Emma, who has been diagnosed with ADHD and anxiety

That, in a nutshell, is the focus of this chapter—just how much lifestyle matters and what you need to know about the impact of sleep, exercise, play, and nutrition on mental health. These tips are for you and your whole family.

## How Sleep Can Improve Mental Health

We tend to treat sleep as an unnecessary frill—something to cut out of our schedules when something has to give (as is too often the case). But a good night's sleep is essential for our mental functioning. Sleep is the time when our brain switches into maintenance and repair mode, processing and reorganizing information that we acquired during the day and storing it in ways that will allow us to draw on it in the future.

Missing out on just a few hours of sleep can take its toll on us very quickly. We become moody and irritable. We have difficulty finding the right words to express what we're thinking and feeling. We struggle to concentrate and to solve problems. Unfortunately, roughly one-third of us are sleep deprived on an ongoing basis (which the Centers for Disease Control and Prevention defines as sleeping for fewer than seven hours each night). And the situation is even grimmer for our kids: a 2006 poll conducted by the National Sleep Foundation found that 87% of high school students in the United States are sleeping far less than the 8 to 10 hours per night recommended for people their age. That's a very alarming finding, given that sleep deprivation in adolescents is associated with poor concentration, poor grades, drowsy-driving incidents, anxiety, depression, thoughts of suicide, and even suicide attempts.

What's on our minds can interfere with our ability to get a good night's sleep. When occasional worries ramp up into something more severe—like an ongoing struggle with anxiety or depression—sleep is almost always affected. Sometimes it's difficult to figure out which came first: the sleep problem or the mental health challenge. People with sleep problems (either sleeping too little or sleeping too much) are more likely to suffer from mental disorders than people who do not experience sleep problems, says the National Sleep Foundation. Likewise, sleep disruption is likely to accompany a mental disorder.

Getting to sleep is only half the battle, as anyone who has struggled with a sleep problem will be quick to tell you. Staying asleep and sleeping restfully are also key elements of a good night's sleep. And they are often nothing more than the stuff of which dreams are made when people are struggling with a mental health challenge or dealing with the fallout of grief. People who are struggling with depression often experience early-morning wakening, and depressed moods can lead to sleep that is neither restful nor restorative. Spending too much time in rapid-eye-movement sleep (REM sleep, the stage of sleep characterized by rapid eye movements and in which dreaming typically occurs) contributes to depression. Antidepressants help to reduce the amount of time spent in REM sleep. Some people notice that they experience more vivid dreams, or even nightmares, after starting an antidepressant. Adolescents with ADHD tend to have difficulty falling asleep, experience restless sleep, and then have difficulty awakening—they may not be fully alert until around noon. It's not exactly the recipe for academic success.

Fortunately, there are plenty of things you can do to prevent or deal with sleep problems. You should start taking steps to address your sleep problem if you are taking 30 minutes or longer to fall asleep, waking repeatedly in the night, or having difficulty getting back to sleep after waking in the night or early morning. In addition to trying some of the lifestyle modifications listed below, you may wish to seek help from a therapist who specializes in mindfulness-based or cognitive-behavioral therapy for insomnia.

### Use Light to Help Regulate Your Body Clock

Your body relies on natural light levels (whether it's dark or light outside) to decide whether it should be manufacturing melatonin (a hormone that is naturally sedating, which your body should be producing at night) or serotonin (the so-called happiness hormone, which plays a role in warding off depression). Going for a 15- to 30-minute walk in the morning sunshine or sitting in front of a full-spectrum light for 15 to 30 minutes in the morning can help to reset your biological clock and restore normal sleeping patterns.

 **NOTE:** Intensive bright light therapy can trigger manic symptoms in some patients with bipolar disorder. Consult with a mental health professional for advice before embarking on treatment.

And, speaking of light, it's important to understand the impact of blue light on sleep quality. Blue light is the type of light emitted by electronic devices. It is also known to affect levels of the sleep-inducing hormone melatonin, wreaking havoc on our circadian rhythm. So a key strategy for safeguarding sleep in an era of almost ubiquitous digital devices is to park those devices somewhere other than the bedroom and to avoid reading from a screen when your body and brain are winding down to go to sleep. This is definitely one of those situations where you'll have to be prepared to walk the walk of good digital sleep hygiene for your kids.

### Relax—At Least Twice a Day

Figure out which relaxation methods work best for you and work them into your daily routine, both during the day and at bedtime. (See Chapter 5 for some suggested techniques.)

### Tweak Your Diet

Too much protein at bedtime can lead to difficulty falling asleep, because high concentrations of protein can interfere with the absorption of serotonin into the brain, leading to high levels of alertness. Likewise, deficiencies in calcium, magnesium, and the B vitamins can also contribute to insomnia.

■ **NOTE:** See the section later in this chapter on nutrition and mental health.

## Exercise

Don't overlook the benefits of exercise in promoting good sleep. Not only will you sleep longer when you're exercising regularly; you'll also benefit from an increase in rejuvenating slow-wave, deep sleep. Just be sure to time that workout so that it works for—and not against—you: 3 to 6 hours before bedtime is ideal, so your body temperature has a chance to return to baseline by the time you want to head to bed, cueing your body that it's time to go to sleep. See the next section of this chapter for more on exercise and mental health.

## Practice Good Sleep Hygiene

Create a sleep-friendly environment. This means making your bedroom comfortable (cool, quiet, dark) and soothing (banish electronics). Avoid heavy meals within 3 hours of bedtime. Limit caffeine intake during the day (particularly within 4 to 6 hours of bedtime) and avoid alcohol before bedtime. Have a warm bath 1 to 2 hours before you go to bed: the drop in body temperature that occurs after a bath will help to cue your body that it's time for sleep. Avoid bright light in the evening—and the blue light from electronics at bedtime—to encourage the production of healthy levels of melatonin. Go to bed and wake up at the same time each day, even on weekends, and limit any daytime naps to a maximum of 15 minutes. Better yet, avoid napping at all.

## Don't Stress Out about Sleep

I know, it's easier said than done, but getting stressed will only make the problem worse. When you're stressed, your body ramps up production of the activating neurotransmitters norepinephrine, epinephrine, and cortisol, which normally subside at night, making it even more difficult for you to obtain the good night's sleep you so desperately crave. Instead of obsessing about the sleep you're not getting (what sleep psychologists refer to as "negative sleep thoughts" or NSTs), replace those NSTs with your own personalized mantra that reflects the reality of your situation, while infusing a bit of calmness and hope. John Arden, author of *Rewire Your Brain: Think*

*Your Way to a Better Life*, suggests the following: "'I might get back to sleep or I might not. Either way, it isn't the end of the world,' 'If I don't get a good night's sleep tonight, I will tomorrow night.'"

# How Exercise Can Improve Mental Health

Exercise boosts our energy. It helps us sleep better. It increases blood flow to the brain, leaving us feeling calmer and more alert. It improves our focus and concentration. It can even boost our self-esteem. It's no wonder physical activity is increasingly becoming part of the prescription for the treatment of depression and anxiety.

So, what is it about exercise that gives it such an impact on our mental health?

Scientists believe there are at least a couple of different mechanisms at work.

### Exercise Improves Mood and Reduces Feelings of Anxiety

Not only does exercise boost endorphins (the body's natural pain relievers and stress fighters); it also helps to balance other neurotransmitters in the brain, including serotonin (which is involved in mood, impulsivity, anger, and aggressiveness), norepinephrine (which is involved in attention, perception, motivation, and arousal), and dopamine (which is involved in learning, reward, attention, and movement). If you happen to be taking an antidepressant drug that affects serotonin, norepinephrine, or epinephrine, your antidepressant will work even better when it's teamed up with regular exercise. It's hard to overstate the impact of exercise on mental health: "Exercise has a profound impact on cognitive abilities and mental health," say John J. Ratey and Eric Hagerman in their book *Spark: The Revolutionary New Science of Exercise and the Brain*. "It is simply one of the best treatments we have for most psychiatric problems."

### Exercise Reduces Stress

Exercise helps to relieve feelings of stress in your body and your mind by reducing muscle tension, bringing down levels of the body's stress hormones (which helps to improve focus and attention), distracting you from your worries, and boosting feelings of resilience and competence (it feels good to be treating your body well). Exercise has been demonstrated to reduce levels of anxiety by as much as 50 percent—and those benefits begin to kick in right from the first workout.

You can help your child enjoy the stress-reducing benefits of physical activity by providing him with opportunities to learn how his body responds to various types of movement. "Patterned, repetitive sensory input such as music, dance, deep breathing, or drumming" can be used to induce relaxation and increase children's capacity to learn, notes Susan E. Craig *in Reaching and Teaching Children Who Hurt:* "Play games where you move with the child from very slow to fast to very fast," she suggests. Combining sound with movement can help your child make the connection between movement and body sensation: "Produce soft voice sounds and then louder sounds and then go from louder to softer," suggests Alice Sterling Honig in *Little Kids, Big Worries: Stress-Busting Tips for Early Childhood Classrooms.*

### Exercise Improves Sleep

Sleep quality improves as you become physically active, leading to a sleep-related boost in mental health. (See the sleep section of this chapter for a discussion of the effects of sleep on mental health.) And as you start sleeping better, you have more energy and motivation to exercise, which in turn leads to more good sleep. It's an upward cycle that can trigger far-reaching health changes.

### Exercise Sparks the Growth of New Brain Cells

This is a game changer for anyone dealing with chronic depression. There's no doubt about it: chronic depression takes a toll on the brain. Studies have shown that the hippocampus (the sea horse–shaped part of the brain that is responsible for storing and retrieving information) can be up to 15 percent smaller in people who are chronically depressed. "In depression, it seems that in certain areas, the brain's ability to adapt grinds to a halt," explain Ratey and Hagerman. "The shutdown in depression is a shutdown of learning at the cellular level. Not only is the brain locked into a negative loop of self-hate, but it also loses the flexibility to work its way out of the hole." Exercise can reverse this process by flooding the brain with neurochemicals and growth factors, leading to an increase in the number of

> The mind is not a vessel to be filled, but a fire to be kindled.
> —Plutarch

neurons in the hippocampus and the number of interconnections between neurons in the hippocampus—something that may make all the difference for a brain that is stuck in the hole of depression.

### Exercise Helps to Counter the Feelings of Hopelessness That Often Accompany Depression

It gives a person struggling with depression a sense of control over her own recovery. "In consciously making the decision to do something for yourself, you begin to realize you can do something for yourself," explain Ratey and Hagerman.

The key to making exercise work for you (at least in terms of your mental health) is to make it part of your life on a regular basis (see the chart below) but without going to boot camp–like extremes, says Arden. "The extremes of no exercise or excessive exercise do not promote a healthy brain," he notes. "Exercise moderately and vigorously."

---

### What Physical Activity Looks Like for People of Various Ages

Children and adolescents ages 6–17 years need at least 1 hour of physical activity each day—and that should include moderate to vigorous aerobic activity (at least 3 days a week) as well as muscle- and bone-strengthening physical activity (at least 3 days a week). That's according to *The Physical Activity Guidelines for Americans,* issued by the U.S. Department of Health and Human Services. But what does physical activity look like for a toddler as opposed to a teen? That's what this chart is all about.

| Age | What physical activity means for people this age |
|---|---|
| **Birth to age 1** | Interactive floor-based play (tummy time, reaching for or grasping balls or other toys), rolling, crawling |
| **Toddlers and preschoolers** | Climbing stairs, moving around the house, playing outside, brisk walking, running, dancing, basically any activity that gets kids moving |
| **School-age children and teens** | Aerobic activities like running or swimming as well as activities that strengthen muscle and bone |

*Sources:* Data from the Centers for Disease Control and Prevention "Youth Physical Activity Guidelines Toolkit" (*www.cdc.gov/healthyschools/physicalactivity/guidelines. htm*) and the Canadian Physical Activity Guidelines (*www.csep.ca/en/guidelines/get-the-guidelines*).

## How Play Can Improve Mental Health

One of the most powerful things we can do for our children's mental health—and our own mental health—is to make more time for play.

In their book *Play: How It Shapes the Brain, Opens the Imagination, and Invigorates the Soul*, Stuart Brown and Christopher Vaughan emphasize the brain-boosting benefits of active play (play that incorporates moderate to vigorous physical activity): "Active play selectively stimulates brain-derived neurotrophic factor (which stimulates nerve growth) in the amygdala (where emotions get processed) and the dorsolateral prefrontal cortex (where executive decisions are processed)."

Brown and Vaughan also stress the social and creative benefits of play: "Play is a way to put us in synch with those around us. It is a way to tap into common emotions and thoughts and share them with others. . . . Creative play takes our minds to places we have never been, pioneering new paths that the real world can follow."

And, of course, where we play is as important as how we play. In his book *Last Child in the Woods*, author and environmentalist Richard Louv, who is best known for coining the phrase "nature-deficit disorder," stresses the importance of providing children with opportunities to play outdoors and of planning activities that include time in nature. "More time in green outdoor settings can reduce symptoms of hyperactivity and attention deficits and improve self-discipline," he notes.

The take-away message is obvious: don't downplay the importance of play. It's the pause that refreshes and replenishes our minds.

## How Nutrition Can Improve Mental Health

If we are what we eat, it's no wonder our mental health has been suffering. The way we eat today is very different from the way our grandparents ate. Our diets are heavily reliant on processed foods as opposed to nutrient-rich whole foods. We're eating fewer fruits and vegetables than ever before—and those fruits and vegetables are being grown in soil that has become increasingly depleted of nutrients over the past 50 years. Just as our intake of key nutrients has been decreasing, our intake of unhealthy fats, salt, sugar, and food additives has been increasing.

What hasn't changed, of course, is what our brains need to function at their best: a healthy balance of complex carbohydrates, essential fats, amino acids from proteins, vitamins and minerals, and water. Here's what you need to know about the role of each of these important nutrients in promoting good mental health.

### Carbohydrates

Not all carbohydrates are created equal—at least when it comes to fueling the brain. When slow-releasing, or complex, carbohydrates (found in foods like whole grains, vegetables, and beans) are digested and then turned into glucose, they provide a steadier and more stable fuel supply than what simple carbohydrates (found in cookies and soda pop) can deliver. Eating carbohydrates also helps to relieve feelings of stress. When you eat carbohydrates, insulin is released into your bloodstream. This insulin proceeds to clear out all of the amino acids in your bloodstream other than tryptophan, which is then free to enter the brain, where it is converted into the feel-good neurotransmitter serotonin. Serotonin reduces pain, decreases appetite, and leaves you feeling calm. It's no wonder many people who are feeling stressed try to self-medicate with carbs.

### Essential Fats

Just as there are good carbs and bad carbs, there are good fats and bad fats. The worst offenders, in terms of messing with brain function, are trans fats (partially hydrogenated oils), liquid vegetable oils that become more solid when hydrogen is added during the manufacturing process. The problem with trans fats is that they end up taking the place of essential fatty acids (EFAs) in the brain without delivering the same nutritional benefits. EFAs cannot be manufactured by the body and so must come directly from food sources. Each type of essential fatty acid plays an important role in the structuring of brain cells (also known as neurons), making smooth communication possible within the brain. Nutritional experts suggest that most people eating Western diets consume too much omega-6 and not enough omega-3. Our unbalanced intake of omega-3 and omega-6 fats has been linked to a number of mental health problems, including depression. "Observational and experimental studies show that diets high in omega 6 fatty acids and low in omega 3 fatty acids contribute to depression, aggression, and [cardiovascular disease]," noted a group of researchers from the Oregon Research Institute in *American Psychologist*. One of the best sources of omega-3 fatty acids is fish. Fish and shellfish that contain higher levels of these fatty acids and are also low in mercury include anchovies, capelin, char, hake, herring, Atlantic mackerel, mullet, pollock (Boston bluefish), salmon, smelts, rainbow trout, lake whitefish, blue crab, shrimp, clams, mussels, and oysters. The U.S. Environmental Protection Agency website (*www.epa.gov*) and the U.S. Food and Drug Administration website (*www.fda.gov*) have detailed information about limiting exposure to mercury while enjoying the benefits of eating fish.

## The Big Four: Four Key Neurotransmitters and How They Are Affected by Food

| Neurotransmitter | What it does | Effects of a deficiency | What can make a deficiency worse | Foods that encourage your body to produce more of this neurotransmitter |
|---|---|---|---|---|
| **Acetylcholine** (derived from the water-soluble vitamin choline) | Regulates attention and concentration | Poor memory, lack of creativity, fewer dreams, increased confusion, forgetfulness, disorganization | Sugar, deep-fried foods, junk food, refined and processed foods, cigarettes, alcohol | Eggs, fish |
| **Serotonin** (derived from the amino acid tryptophan) | Regulates mood, well-being, and sleep patterns | Depression, insomnia | Alcohol | Fish, fruit, eggs, avocado, wheat germ, low-fat cheese, lean poultry *Note:* Carbohydrates increase the availability of tryptophan by easing its entry into the brain. |
| **Dopamine** (derived from the amino acid tyrosine) | Controls the brain's pleasure and reward centers; improves mental and physical performance under stress | Lack of motivation, lack of enthusiasm, cravings for stimulants | Caffeinated foods and beverages | Vitamin C–rich fruits and vegetables, wheat germ |
| **GABA** (gamma-aminobutyric acid) | Inhibits excessive brain activity and anxiety | Anxiety, irritability, tension, self-criticism | Sugar, alcohol, caffeinated foods and beverages | Dark green vegetables, seeds and nuts, potatoes, bananas, eggs |

*Sources:* Data from a similar chart in *Feeding Minds: The Impact of Food on Mental Health* (London: Mental Health Foundation, 2006).

### Amino Acids from Protein

Neurotransmitters, the brain's messengers, are created from amino acids. Some amino acids can be manufactured by the body. Other amino acids— the so-called essential amino acids—need to come directly from food sources. If the body isn't able to obtain adequate quantities of these essential amino acids, deficiencies in key neurotransmitters may arise, resulting in mental health challenges and other types of brain dysfunction (see the chart "The Big Four" on page 157). Eating protein-rich foods promotes alertness.

### Vitamins and Minerals

Vitamins and minerals perform important housekeeping functions, converting carbohydrates into glucose, fatty acids into brain cells, and amino acids into neurotransmitters. And some function as antioxidants, protecting the brain from cell-damaging oxidants from food, smoking, alcohol, and stress. When we experience deficiencies in key vitamins and minerals (see the chart "How Deficiencies of Specific Nutrients Affect Mental Health" on pages 159–160), mental health problems may arise.

### Water

Even mild dehydration affects brain functioning, resulting in restless or irritable behavior, loss of concentration, weakness, and feeling unwell.

## What You Can Do

So what can you do to "let food be thy medicine and medicine be thy food," as Hippocrates said so long ago?

### Pay Attention to the Types of Foods
### That Your Family Is Eating

Some foods, like coffee, offer a quick fix, making us feel good over the short term, but can create a bigger problem over the long term if consumed in excess, by causing our brains to become less sensitive to their own signals and less able to produce healthy patterns of brain activity. Other foods, like fried foods, add to the number of cell-damaging oxidants in our brains. And still others—the foods we want to build our diets around (like fruits

# How Deficiencies of Specific Nutrients Affect Mental Health

| Nutrient | Food sources of this nutrient | How deficiencies of this nutrient affect mental health |
| --- | --- | --- |
| **Vitamin B$_1$** (thiamine) | Pork, fish, beans, lentils, nuts, rice, wheat germ | Poor concentration, poor attention |
| **Vitamin B$_2$** (riboflavin) | Dairy products, meat and fish, eggs, mushrooms, almonds, leafy greens, legumes | Depression |
| **Vitamin B$_3$** (niacin) | Whole grains, vegetables | Depression |
| **Vitamin B$_5$** (pantothenic acid) | Whole grains, vegetables | Poor memory, stress |
| **Vitamin B$_6$** (pyridoxine) | Fish, beef, poultry, potatoes, legumes, spinach | Irritability, poor memory, stress, depression |
| **Vitamin B$_9$** (folate) | Green leafy vegetables, lentils, orange juice, bananas | Depression, psychosis |
| **Vitamin B$_{12}$** (cobalamin) | Fish, mollusks (oysters, mussels, and clams), meat, dairy products | Depression, irritability, agitation, psychosis, and obsessive symptoms |
| **Vitamin C** | Citrus fruits, potatoes, tomatoes | Irritability, depression |
| **Vitamin D\*** | Fish, eggs, other foods fortified with vitamin D, including milk | Depression |
| **Vitamin E** | Almonds, sunflower seeds, leafy greens, wheat germ | Depression |
| **Iron** | Beef, chicken, turkey, pork, fish, and shellfish; iron-fortified breads and cereals; spinach; chickpeas, beans, and lentils; dried fruit; tofu | Fatigue, behavior problems |

*One of the best ways to obtain vitamin D is through exposure to sunshine. That can be a challenge during certain times of the year, depending on how far north you live, but do try to take advantage of sunny days when we have them. Even 10 to 15 minutes of sunshine a day can make a big difference.

| Nutrient | Food sources of this nutrient | How deficiencies of this nutrient affect mental health |
| --- | --- | --- |
| Magnesium | Green vegetables, nuts, seeds | Irritability, insomnia, depression |
| Selenium | Wheat germ, brewer's yeast, liver, fish, eggs, garlic, sunflower seeds, Brazil nuts, whole grains | Irritability, depression |
| Zinc | Oysters, nuts, seeds, fish | Confusion, depression, loss of appetite, lack of motivation |

*Note.* Excess intake of vitamin A (which is found in beef liver, dairy products, eggs, carrots, sweet potatoes, and leafy greens) can lead to symptoms of depression.

*Sources:* Data from *Feeding Minds: The Impact of Food on Mental Health* (London: Mental Health Foundation, 2006); National Heart, Lung, and Blood Institute, "How Is Iron-Deficiency Anemia Treated?" (November 6, 2013; *http://www.nhlbi.nih.gov/health/health-topics/topics/ida/treatment.html*); Sue Penckofer, Joanne Kouba, Mary Byrn, and Carol Estwing Ferrans, "Vitamin D and Depression: Where Is All the Sunshine?," *Issues in Mental Health Nursing, 31*(6), 385–393 (2010); Drew Ramsey and Philip R. Muskin, "Vitamin Deficiencies and Mental Health: How Are They Linked?," *Current Psychiatry, 12*(1) (January 2013).

and vegetables that are rich in antioxidants)—nourish and replenish the brain, boosting our mood and mental functioning. And there is growing evidence that a Mediterranean-style diet (a diet that focuses on vegetables, fresh and dried fruits, whole-grain cereals, nuts and legumes, and a moderate amount of red wine) promotes good mental health.

### Make Sure You're Consuming Enough Fruits and Vegetables

Most Americans aren't. A 2015 study by the Centers for Disease Control and Prevention (CDC) found that fewer than 15% of Americans manage to consume the two to four servings of fruit and three to five servings of vegetables each day recommended by the U.S. Department of Agriculture (USDA) *Food Guide Pyramid*. Likewise, an earlier 2014 CDC study found that just 40% of children are getting enough fruit and just 7% are getting enough vegetables.

To get maximum nutritional mileage out of those veggie servings, try to eat a dark-green vegetable (such as broccoli, asparagus, or romaine lettuce) and an orange vegetable (such as carrots or sweet potatoes) every day.

## Go (for) Fish

Americans typically consume about 3.5 ounces of fish per week—just half of what the USDA recommends. In addition to being an excellent source of essential fatty acids, fish delivers brain-friendly selenium, magnesium, and iron. The U.S. Environmental Protection Agency website (*www.epa.gov*) and the U.S. Food and Drug Administration website (*www.fda.gov*) have detailed information about limiting exposure to mercury while enjoying the benefits of eating fish.

## Understand How the Timing and Makeup of Meals and Snacks Affect Mood

Going too long without food leads to dips in blood sugar, which makes mood swings, irritability, and fatigue worse. Likewise, what makes up a meal can also have a major impact on how you feel an hour or two after you've eaten. You'll still have energy left after a meal made up of protein and complex carbohydrates (tuna on whole-grain bread), whereas your blood sugar will be spiking and crashing after a meal made up of simple carbs (a muffin and a bagel), sending your mood spiraling downward with it.

## Figure Out Which Foods Are Likely to Have the Greatest Impact in Terms of Easing Your Child's Symptoms

While we still have much to learn, researchers are beginning to accumulate evidence about the ways in which nutrition can improve the mental health of people living with various types of disorders. Most of this evidence relates to the following types of disorders: anxiety disorders, autism spectrum disorders, ADHD, bipolar disorder, schizophrenia and related disorders, and trauma. See the chart "Nutrition and Mental Health" on pages 162–163. It's important to keep in mind, however, that nutrition is just one piece of the puzzle. In other words, there isn't enough evidence about the impact of good nutrition on mental health to suggest that nutrition should be considered a replacement for other forms of treatment like medication or therapy.

## Be Alert to the Warning Signs of an Eating Disorder

Children and youth who have been diagnosed with mood disorders, anxiety disorders, or substance abuse disorders face an increased risk of developing eating disorders. If your child has received one of these diagnoses, it's important to be alert to the warning signs of eating disorders such as

## Nutrition and Mental Health

| Type of disorder | Nutrition-related issues |
|---|---|
| Anxiety disorders | • Sensory concerns as well as food-specific phobias may result in restricted food choices.<br>• Increased intake of omega-3 through diet (to 3 grams per day) may be helpful in easing symptoms of anxiety. |
| Autism spectrum disorder | • Diet may be lacking in dairy, fiber, calcium, iron, and vitamins D and E. Sensory concerns and difficulty with change may restrict food choices.<br>• Increased intake of omega-3 (especially docosahexaenoic acid, or DHA) through diet (1 to 3 grams per day) may be helpful in easing some symptoms in some individuals.<br>• Evidence is limited regarding the benefits of gluten-free, casein-free diets. |
| ADHD | • Deficiencies of polyunsaturated fatty acids, essential fatty acids, zinc, magnesium, and iron are common.<br>• Iron, magnesium, and zinc supplementation may be helpful.<br>• A gluten-free diet can improve behavior in individuals with ADHD who also have celiac disease.<br>• An additive-free diet (no food coloring or preservatives) may improve symptoms in children who are sensitive to such additives, but such a diet needs to be supervised by a registered dietitian.<br>• Removing sugar from the diet will not improve symptoms of hyperactivity. |
| Bipolar disorder | • Large amounts of sugar, caffeine, and food may be consumed during periods of mania, or there may be times when no food is consumed.<br>• Selenium, folic acid (folate), omega-3 fatty acids, and tryptophan may be helpful in keeping moods stable. Attempts should be made to obtain these nutrients from food sources before resorting to supplements.<br>• Supplementation with 1 to 3 grams of omega-3 fatty acids daily may ease depressive episodes.<br>• People with bipolar disorder are susceptible to celiac disease. If celiac disease is confirmed, a gluten-free diet is recommended. |

| **Depressive disorders** | • Both undereating and overeating may be a problem.<br>• The risk of depression increases with low intakes of omega-3 fatty acids, fruits, and vegetables, and a high intake of refined sugar and processed foods.<br>• Folate (with vitamin $B_{12}$) and omega-3 fatty acid (eicosapentaenoic acid and docosahexaenoic acid) supplementation may be beneficial.<br>• People with depressive disorders are susceptible to celiac disease. If celiac disease is confirmed, a gluten-free diet is recommended. |
|---|---|
| **Schizophrenia and related disorders** | • Diet may be lacking in fruits and vegetables, fiber, vitamin C, and beta carotene.<br>• Individuals who experience hallucinations related to smell and taste may no longer experience pleasure from eating or may have difficulty avoiding health risks associated with eating spoiled food.<br>• Celiac disease is twice as common in people with schizophrenia. If celiac disease is confirmed, a gluten-free diet is recommended.<br>• Omega-3 fatty acid supplementation has not been proven beneficial for people with schizophrenia.<br>• Antipsychotic medications may contribute to weight gain and metabolic disturbance. |
| **Trauma** | • Sensory issues, hyperarousal, being easily startled, and feelings of numbness (all effects of trauma) can affect appetite and eating.<br>• Foods rich in antioxidants (vegetables, fruit, whole grains, beans, lentils, nuts, seeds, vegetable oils, garlic, green tea) may help to counteract the effects of stress. |

*Sources*: Data from Royal College of Psychiatrists, "Eating Well and Mental Health, (November 6, 2013; *www.rcpsych.ac.uk/healthadvice/problemsdisorders/ eatingwellandmentalhealth.aspx*); Mental Health Foundation, *Feeding Minds: The Impact of Food on Mental Health* (London: 2006); Dietitians of Canada, *Promoting Mental Health Through Healthy Eating and Nutritional Care* (December 2012).

anorexia, bulimia, or binge-eating disorder. Some of the warning signs include:

- Distorted body image
- Intense fear of being fat
- Strenuous exercise
- Hoarding and hiding food
- Secret eating and/or heading to the bathroom immediately after eating
- Extreme food restriction
- Sleep disruption
- Physical deterioration (for example, feeling cold all the time, difficulty sleeping)
- Injuries associated with the eating disorder, such as cuts and calluses across the top of the finger joints (the result of sticking fingers down the throat to induce vomiting)

If you notice some of these symptoms in your child, express your concern in a calm and caring way, validate your child's feelings, and seek medical attention for your child. For more about the diagnosis and treatment of eating disorders, please visit the National Eating Disorders Association website (*nationaleatingdisorders.org*).

### Understand How Caffeine Affects Mood

Caffeine may seem like your best friend when you're feeling dragged out and depressed, but it's actually more like a frenemy. While it may give you that quick energy fix you're craving, it can also leave you feeling anxious, cause sleep problems, and leave you feeling even more depressed over the long run. To make matters worse, it acts as a diuretic (a substance that promotes the production of urine), so it tends to dehydrate you—and dehydration further increases your feelings of fatigue. Some friend, huh?

   While you might shudder at the mere idea of ever parting ways with this BFF, I parted ways with caffeine about 5 years ago—and it was the first crucial step in regaining control over my physical and mental health. It's worth thinking about how caffeine is affecting your life—or your child's life—and considering more sustainable alternatives to the coffee, cola, or chocolate energy fix.

## Understand How Alcohol Affects the Brain

Our culture may tell us that alcohol is an essential ingredient in the recipe for having fun, but it's bad news for anyone struggling with a mental health problem. Alcohol is a depressant, so it brings down your mood. That's what it's biochemically designed to do. It also robs your body of important nutrients that your brain requires to ward off depression and other mental health problems. (Your liver has to draw on thiamine, zinc, and other nutrients during the alcohol detoxification process.) Your best bet is to abstain from alcohol if you can. If your child is the one who is struggling, it's important to talk to your child about the impact of alcohol on mental health and how alcohol affects any medications that have been prescribed, so that he can make an informed decision about these issues too.

## Look at the Big Picture

Don't overlook the possibility that a nutritional deficiency or other physical health problem could be contributing to your child's symptoms. Iron deficiency, blood sugar irregularities, and thyroid problems can result in mood and anxiety disorder symptoms.

## Seek Help in Dealing with Any Issues That Are Interfering with Your Child's Eating

Sometimes children who are struggling with mental health disorders exhibit specific eating-related behaviors that can make it difficult for them to settle down to eat a meal or to consume adequate nutrients (see the chart on healthy eating on page 166). If you are finding it difficult to work through these issues with your child, it is important to seek professional assistance from a registered dietitian, a therapist, and/or an occupational therapist.

As you can see in the chart, lifestyle matters a lot when it comes to mental health. Whether you're looking to prevent mental health problems or to deal with an existing issue, there's always room for (lifestyle) improvement. Tackling these types of changes as a family, or with support from a friend who is also interested in making changes, makes it easier. Start small (commit to increasing the number of glasses of water you drink or the number of steps you take in a day), and then find ways to keep building on those initial successes. See the official website for this book, *www.anndouglas.net*, for additional resources to support you on the journey to better health.

## How to Troubleshoot Specific Emotional and Behavioral Issues That May Interfere with Healthy Eating

| Problem | Possible solutions |
| --- | --- |
| **Your child finds it difficult to settle down to eat a meal because of anxiety or restlessness.** | • Offer small, frequent meals and snacks.<br>• Offer one type of food at a time (and possibly one type of utensil at a time).<br>• Limit caffeine.<br>• Consider nutritional supplements. |
| **Your child avoids certain foods or food groups as a result of obsessive thoughts about food.** | • Offer small, frequent meals and snacks.<br>• Consider nutritional supplements.<br>• Avoid caffeine as it worsens anxiety. |
| **Your child uses food to soothe feelings of anxiety, leading to overeating.** | • Have healthy, lower-calorie foods on hand.<br>• Avoid caffeine as it worsens anxiety. |
| **Your child is sensitive to certain textures and consistencies and avoids certain foods as a result.** | • Modify the textures of foods and beverages as needed. |
| **Your child is having trouble sleeping and is hungrier than usual as a result.** | • Avoid caffeinated food and drink as well as high-fat or spicy foods within 8 hours of bedtime.<br>• Encourage low-calorie evening snacks if nighttime snacking is a concern. |
| **Your child's appetite increases and decreases as she experiences highs and lows in mood.** | • Offer regular meals and snacks in order to minimize blood sugar fluctuations. |

*Source*: Data from Dietitians of Canada, *Promoting Mental Health Through Healthy Eating and Nutritional Care* (December 2012).

# Part IV

# Your Community

We human beings are social creatures. We rely on relationships with others to thrive. And yet when a child is struggling with a mental health, neurodevelopmental, or behavioral challenge, relationships can start to break down. In this next part of the book you'll read about the importance of creating community for yourself and your child—supports that may serve as anchors in the storm.

Going to school and making friends are experiences that most children take for granted. But if you have a child who is struggling with a psychiatric disorder, these goals can become major sources of stress. Chapter 10 offers ways you can work with your child's teacher to make school a more positive and less stressful experience, providing advice on what to ask for and how to ask. In Chapter 11, you'll find strategies for helping your child learn how to make friends, a skill that doesn't necessarily come quickly or easily to all children.

Your child isn't the only one who would benefit from some additional support during this difficult time. That's why, in Chapter 12, I talk about what you can do to enlarge your own circle of support, both by connecting with other parents who understand the challenges you are facing and by finding allies at work.

You don't have to face the storm alone, and neither does your child. You can reach out to your community for the support you need to weather the challenges ahead.

# 10

# Working with
# Your Child's School

School plays a major role in our children's lives, providing them with opportunities to learn and grow socially, emotionally, and academically. That said, if a child is struggling with a mental health disorder, school may become an experience to be endured rather than enjoyed—assuming a child is able to function well enough to continue attending school at all. (Not everyone can.)

In this chapter, I'll be talking about the types of issues that can arise at school for your child, as well as ways you can work with your child's school to try to address those issues.

> Be proactive and do what we did: work with the school while you lead the process.
> —Lyn, mother of Ben, who has been diagnosed with ADHD

## The Types of Difficulties
## Your Child Might Be Experiencing at School

Mental health challenges affect a child's thinking, emotions, and behavior. They can have far-reaching impacts on her ability to function at school.

Depending on the nature and severity of the problems, your child might be having difficulty with any of the following:

- Getting up for school in the morning or staying awake in class
- Concentrating

- Filtering out background noise and other distractions
- Making sense of verbal instructions
- Switching from one task to another during the school day
- Approaching the teacher for help with classroom assignments
- Initiating conversations with or maintaining relationships with peers
- Prioritizing tasks to meet deadlines (or breaking individual tasks into chunks to get started and stay on track when working on a big project)
- Tolerating interruptions or changes in plans
- Coping with negative feedback
- Solving problems and coping with day-to-day frustrations
- Coping with overwhelming emotions
- Finding the motivation or the energy required to cope with the demands of school
- Completing homework

When things start to go wrong at school, they tend to spiral downward very quickly. Christine recalls how the situation played out for her family prior to her son Will's diagnosis with severe ADHD and an anxiety disorder. "In the first grade, Will was sent home from school about once a week. His teacher simply didn't know how to deal with him and so would send him home. We hoped second grade, with a different teacher, would be better. Unfortunately, he was suspended in second grade. . . . Will was miserable at school. He was constantly being disciplined, reprimanded, and sent home. He was becoming socially isolated and depressed. His grades were also suffering, and he often told me that he thought he was the stupidest kid in his class."

Dealing with the school system is a major source of stress for parents raising children with psychiatric disorders or neurodevelopmental challenges. Studies have shown that these children are more likely to be suspended than other children, and that students with ADHD or behavioral disorders are particularly likely to be suspended.

Meg can relate to that experience. Her son, Jayden, who has been diagnosed with an anxiety disorder but likely also has an autism spectrum disorder, has experienced considerable struggles at school. "Every day we would cross our fingers he could make it through the day without a phone call to pick him up. The days that we would receive a call to pick him up because they could not manage him were the most difficult. Those were the days we felt concerned, scared, and defeated. It wasn't a good situation for the school, for us as parents, and mostly for Jayden.

"We understood that Jayden's unique way of thinking and learning would pose difficulties in his school journey. What shocked us was his response to a situation that he wasn't comfortable with. He went into fight-or-flight mode. He no longer used the cognitive part of his brain but would respond instead with impulsive and sometimes violent behavior. This terrified us. We never imagined our sweet boy, who wouldn't even squish an ant, acting in a violent manner at school—pushing a teacher, principal, or education assistant or destroying a room. I spent many evenings crying, wondering what to do and how to help Jayden. I was able to take my anger and frustration and channel those feelings into compassion and creative ideas to help. I realized that it didn't feel good for Jayden to be losing control. In fact, he would feel guilty and sad about hurting and disappointing people. I realized it was time for me to start focusing on identifying his triggers and looking for ways to help Jayden manage his 'big' feelings."

## First Things First:
## Know Your Child's Rights

One of the most powerful things you can do to increase your ability to advocate on your child's behalf at school is to understand your child's rights under three key pieces of federal legislation: the Individuals with Disabilities Education Act (IDEA), the Americans with Disabilities Act (ADA), and Section 504 of the Rehabilitation Act. The IDEA guarantees each child the right to a free appropriate public education that meets her needs for education and related services in the "least restrictive environment" possible.* The ADA prohibits discrimination against individuals with disabilities in a wide range of settings, including both public and private schools. And Section 504 of the Rehabilitation Act protects the rights of individuals with disabilities in programs and activities that receive funding from the U.S. Department of Education, spelling out, in a so-called 504 plan, the accommodations that need to be made for a student whose disability "substantially" limits his ability to participate in school.

---

*While the IDEA was not designed to address the needs of students attending private schools, there are situations in which its provisions apply to them. If a public school decides that it is necessary to place your child in a private special education school to meet its commitments as defined by your child's IEP, then the public school continues to be responsible for ensuring that the private school implements the IEP. It is also worth reiterating that private schools are bound by the provisions of Section 504 and may be required to provide modifications, accommodations, and access to educational opportunities. Depending on the nature of your child's disabilities and the educational options available to you in your community, it might be worth consulting with a special education consultant and/or an attorney who specializes in education law so that you're clear up front about your child's rights.

Exactly what these rights and protections mean in practical terms can vary from state to state and even county to county—and parents are often the ones required to do the hard work of making the school system work for their child. In a perfect world, taking a collaborative approach to dealing with your child's school would be all that is required to start to make things better for your child. Concerns would be flagged by you or the school; a psychoeducational assessment would be conducted; and your child's needs would be noted and addressed in an IEP developed in collaboration with the school. That's how things are supposed to play out, but, unfortunately, things can get a little bogged down in the real world, in which case super-human patience and even stronger advocacy skills may be required. That's what this next section of the chapter is all about—helping you figure out how to make complex legislation and an admittedly imperfect system work for your child and your family.

## Working with Your Child's Teachers

Teachers—like schools—vary tremendously in terms of their ability to meet the needs of students who are facing types of challenges. So choosing the right school and finding the right teachers can make a huge difference for your child—assuming, of course, that you have the luxury of choice. (Not everyone does. Depending on where you live, there may not be any workable alternatives to sending your child to the local school, for reasons of geography and/or finances. And, if that's the case, it's important to both accept that reality *and* do your best to try to make things better for your child.) But assuming that you do have a little wiggle room—you have the option of sending your child to a different school or you're able to work with your child's school to modify her classroom environment or to ensure that she's placed with a teacher who is up to the challenge of meeting her needs, for example—you have the potential to make a very big difference for your child.

If you *do* have the ability to choose your child's school (as opposed to having to settle for the only available option by default), you will want to spend some time thinking about what you're looking for in a school *before* you start scheduling school visits. You'll save yourself a lot of legwork by zeroing in on those schools that meet your key criteria (for example, the school's educational approach, discipline policies, and its ability to offer appropriate accommodations, modifications, and supports to someone with your child's particular needs). Then, when you schedule your school visits, you can focus on what really matters: Will your child be able to be successful in this environment? And will he feel supported and accepted?

Sometimes, despite your best efforts, your child may end up in a school situation that is less than ideal—to put it mildly. That has certainly been Laura's family's experience. Her son Gabriel has been diagnosed with Asperger syndrome (now diagnosed simply as autism spectrum disorder in DSM-5) and exhibits a lot of OCD-type behaviors. She explains: "We were able to access wonderful, quality services [at the first school Gabriel attended], and I believe that some of that work absolutely changed the trajectory of his life. Throughout preschool and kindergarten, he received intensive one-on-one therapy a couple of afternoons each week, and it made a huge difference in his communication skills. Then we moved to [another part of the country] when Gabriel was in first grade. I found that the school there really underestimated his abilities. They encouraged us to put him in a remedial program, which we refused to do. At one meeting the psychologist for the school board essentially scolded me for making decisions that she believed weren't based on Gabriel's needs but my own! And then it turned out that she was looking at the wrong file: she wasn't talking about Gabriel at all. When we had to move again after second grade (my husband was in the military at the time), the teacher said that we would be doing incredible damage to Gabriel by moving him around and that I should refuse to move with my husband.

"In third grade, Gabriel had the best teacher he is likely to ever have. This young man saw nothing but potential in Gabriel and worked tirelessly to access services through the school board for him . . . Gabriel made tremendous progress that year.

"We've had good and not-so-good experiences since then, and it mostly comes down to the quality of the teaching. Some teachers are amazing and some are mediocre. We've only had one or two 'bad' teachers."

Here's the good news: You may not win the teacher lottery every year, but in most cases you'll be able to establish a working relationship that will allow you to make things better for your child. It also doesn't hurt to have a conversation with the principal ahead of time about which teacher

I've lived in a tiny Kansas town for 10 years because the school system here is phenomenal. They know Jess, they care about Jess, they try to give Jess everything she needs. So as much as I hate living in a tiny Kansas town, that's just the deal I made. I know people who sue school districts and so on, and I just don't think there's enough time for that. If you can't get what your child needs without a huge struggle, you need to do something drastic like move into a different school district. There is just so little room for error.

—Jennifer, mother of Jessica, who experiences a variety of physical and mental health difficulties related to her tuberous sclerosis diagnosis might be the best fit for your child for the upcoming school year—a teacher who understands your child's challenge and who will work with you to put the necessary supports in place.

Here are a few tips on forging a healthy working alliance with your child's teacher.

### Try to Get to Know Your Child's Teacher(s) as Early as Possible during the School Year

You might be able to make a connection even sooner than that—at the end of the previous school year or just before school starts. You want the teacher to head into the new school year knowing you're eager to work with her to help both your child and the teacher have a successful year.

### Inspire Your Child's Teacher(s) to Become Curious about Who Your Child Is as a Person

"As an educator myself, I know there is a stigma associated with a diagnosis and a resulting IEP with a behavioral exceptionality," says Leigh, whose son, Skyler, has been diagnosed with ADHD, anxiety, and depression. "Unless someone bothers to read the documentation and truly attempts to understand my son, they might dismiss him as a problem child without ever really knowing that much of what he demonstrates is a response to real, authentic fear. I have become a proactive advocate on my son's behalf to help people understand him, to know what are best practice strategies, and to provide support for the folks who work with him in a school setting." Educator Bev Ogilvie, author of *ConnectZone.org: Building Connectedness in Schools*, believes that forging healthy relationships with caring adults is key to the success of students. "Kids are relational learners. . . . To support the mental health of students, we need to walk the talk of connectedness. This means nurturing meaningful connections between students, staff, parents and community members. It means nurturing a health-promoting school environment in which we strive to ensure that students feel safe from physical and emotional harm, secure in their relationships with teachers and peers, and valued as important members of their school."

### Ask Questions

The following types of questions will help to convey to the teacher(s) that you are hoping you can work together to help make things better for your child:

- "What can I do to support the work you are doing with my child in the classroom?"
- "What are some ways I can support my child's learning at home?"
- "What are the best time and the best way for me to get in touch with you?"

The rewards of taking a team approach to dealing with your child's challenges at school can be considerable, says Kim, whose son, Tom, has been diagnosed with ADHD as well as a learning disability. "Tom's school has been a great support throughout his elementary years. He took breaks (either at his own initiative or with a little encouragement from his teachers) and learned some good self-advocacy and calming skills as well. I believe that Tom has done so well in school because we have all worked well as a team to support him."

### Ask for the Teacher's Help

Forging a relationship that is collaborative rather than combative can reap major dividends for your child. Heather, mother of four children, all of whom have faced some sort of struggle, remembers one meeting where a school psychologist was starting to dig in her heels on a particular issue— and how Heather managed to turn that resistance into cooperation: "I knew she wasn't going to budge as long as I was pushing her, so instead, I shifted tactics: I asked for her help, tapped into her expertise, and suddenly she was coming up with a list of accommodations for our son to select from."

Heather was also amazed by the amount of practical assistance and support her children's school was willing to offer in the absence of an official diagnosis: "[One of our children's] teachers called a meeting, and we talked about what was going on, and they said they didn't care if he had a diagnosis or not; that they would provide whatever accommodations made sense to get him through it." It was an incredibly emotional moment for Heather: "I cried," she recalls. For her, it felt like the system was working as it should work for children who are struggling: "They saw the same things we saw [in Michael], and they were willing to do whatever was required to help him achieve at his highest potential."

### Keep the Conversation Going

"You have got to get everyone, including the principal, in a room together at least once a semester," says Jennifer. And, of course, you'll want to keep the lines of communication open in between those face-to-face meetings, either by writing in your child's home–school communication notebook or by emailing or text messaging the teacher directly (whatever works best for all concerned).

### Identify Other Potential Allies at School

Don't overlook the impact that other staff members, including support staff, can have on your child's ability to function well at school. Cheyenne has found, for example, that forging an alliance with the receptionists in the school office has made it possible for her daughter, Keisha, who struggles with ADHD and anxiety, to work through moments of crisis when she would otherwise have to be sent home from school. She explains: "The receptionists have been amazing. If Keisha shows up in the office crying, they will stop what they're doing and help resolve her problem." Her advice to other parents? "You have to find an advocate at school—someone who really cares for your kid and really gets your kid. . . . And you have to make a plan with those people for whatever situations could arise at school. That makes all the difference."

### Ensure That Your Child's IEP Is Rich in Strategies and Practical Accommodations

You should be invited to provide input into the IEP while it is being created and to comment on (and not just rubber-stamp) the resulting product. You should also be invited to participate in future meetings to monitor your child's progress and to assist with the process of updating the IEP. The IEP that is created for your child as a result of that process of collaboration should:

- List areas of strength, areas of weakness, and goals for your child.
- Specify the strategies that will be used to help your child achieve these goals.
- Detail the methods that will be used to track your child's progress toward these goals.
- Note the types of services and resources that will be made available to your child.
- Indicate how the curriculum will be adapted or modified for your child.

Some of the types of supports and accommodations that have worked well for students include:

- Allowing the student to sit at the front of the classroom to minimize distractions
- Providing the student with noise-canceling headphones to eliminate background noise
- Placing tennis balls on the feet of chairs to reduce noise levels in the classroom
- Providing the student with sensory tools (such as squishy balls, vibrating pens, chewable pencil toppers, or fidget toys) that allow him to control his level of stimulation, thereby achieving his optimal level of focus required for learning and socialization
- Providing the student with opportunities to move her body while she's learning (for example, providing a Movin' Sit cushion—an inflatable wedge that allows for movement during seatwork and also assists with posture and concentration)
- Having the teacher cue the student when it's time to refocus attention (for example, if important instructions about an assignment are about to be provided)
- Teaching the student how to break assignments down into more manageable steps and having the teacher check in on progress frequently
- Providing the student with a full set of notes for all classes plus a set of textbooks for use at home
- Offering the student technical assistance (for example, access to technology in the classroom) if associated learning disabilities or side effects from medications make writing by hand difficult
- Scheduling assignments and tests so that due dates fall throughout the course as opposed to within a concentrated period of time
- Providing the student with the option of heading for a safe place within the school if the student needs to regain emotional control (typically, the student and the teacher agree on a signal that can be used to indicate that the student is going to head to the safe place to take a break)
- Providing the student with a place to go during recess where he can relax and connect with an adult if he needs a break from peer social relationships
- Providing the student with advance warning if it's necessary to make changes to the daily schedule or the usual classroom routine (even a brief heads-up can make a big difference)
- Encouraging the student to use coping techniques (self-distraction, relaxation breathing, positive self-talk) if she is becoming stressed or agitated

- Providing the student with opportunities to work on any assigned homework during the school day so he doesn't have to spend a lot of time at night working on homework
- Giving the student as much notice as possible of assignment due dates so that she can plan ahead and schedule any extra help needed to complete the assignment
- Offering the student extra time for writing tests as well as the option of writing tests in a distraction-free environment
- Providing the student with access to an educational assistant and other sources of support in the school (for example, appointments with a school counselor or social worker)
- Offering the student the option to attend school on a part-time basis or to pursue other alternative learning arrangements (such as home tutoring, placement in a specialized alternative school, or distance learning)
- Providing enhanced communication between home and school (via weekly check-in phone calls or a daily communication book that is sent back and forth between home and school) and adequate briefing of substitute teachers about the supports and accommodations the student requires to be successful at school

**NOTE:** Here's one final thing you need to know about IEPs: An IEP is a living document rather than a static, unchanging document. It is meant to evolve and change along with your child's circumstances and needs. This is why it needs to be reviewed and updated regularly (at least once a year).

## Working Through the Tough Stuff

It's important to maintain a solutions-oriented focus with your child's teacher(s) and others at your child's school, even when the going gets tough. You'll find this easier to do if you keep conversations focused on your ultimate goal: making things better for your child.

This isn't always easy to do. You may find that you require superhuman patience (or a superstrong support network—see Chapter 12) to continue to advocate on behalf of your child when you feel like you're being faced with seemingly endless roadblocks and delays. But it's worth it to try to troubleshoot problems if you can.

Sometimes it's a matter of trying to see the world through the eyes of your child's teacher—to understand the roadblocks she may be encountering on a day-to-day basis, no matter how hardworking or well-meaning she may be. "Teachers get a lot of heat, and some of them absolutely deserve it," explains Jennifer, mother of Jessica. "But most of them are doing their best. If you listen, you'll learn what is constraining them. Sometimes it's laws or regulations. Sometimes it's a lack of vision. If you know why you're having a problem, it's easier to solve that problem."

Sometimes the problem you're facing is bigger than you or the school. You've run up against a problem with the school system that is preventing your child from receiving the educational supports he both needs and deserves. In this case, you may need to seek advice from an educational consultant and/or an attorney who specializes in educational law to lobby for your child's rights within the system. This is the route that Linda and her family ended up taking, repeatedly, to secure appropriate supports for her son, Sam, who struggles with ADHD and learning disabilities. She explains: "We hired an attorney who specializes in educational law to convince our local school district that their programs for kids like Sam were insufficient and that they were obligated to fund him in a private school. Eventually we had success. [Then] Sam's emotional disabilities (mental health issues) overwhelmed his learning disabilities and he was asked to leave his LD school. It was difficult to find an appropriate school in our area for children with emotional disabilities. We worked with private (expensive) consultants to identify other placements and then struggled to get our school district to fund them, eventually successfully."

Sometimes you simply have to accept the fact that some schools—and school boards—still have a long way to go when it comes to meeting the needs of students who are struggling with mental health and development challenges. You can—and should—continue to advocate for change but, for the sake of your sanity, you might also want to accept the fact that things aren't likely to change dramatically anytime soon. (You can do both: accept what is while continuing to push for what's possible.) Just understand that the emotional toll on you, the parent of a child whose needs aren't being met particularly well by the school system, can be considerable.

Tami finds herself dealing with a lot of emotions as a result of the struggles her son Adam has faced at school. "I have felt rage, frustration, and deep sadness—particularly when the school has not been able to handle Adam's behavior," she explains. "I get angry that there isn't better funding for special needs, frustrated that (some) teachers don't really 'get' what it means to have ADHD, and sad about the difficulties Adam has to go through every single day, not just because of the condition itself but because others don't know how to help him."

Rebecca resents the fact that she is having to provide her daughter's teacher with a crash course in managing anxiety in children—information she expected the teacher to have. She explains: "I met with Madalyn's teacher on Monday morning, and I feel like I'm arming her with information that all teachers should know, like what childhood anxiety looks like or how to accommodate Madalyn in usual classroom activities. For instance, when it comes to tests, Madalyn should have more time or fewer questions. And yet I find myself having to remind an education professional why she needs these accommodations."

Leigh also recalls feeling let down by some of the teachers at her son's school. "At home, our greatest gains came from using collaborative problem solving, because we felt this would give Skyler the skills to work through relationship challenges. The issue we encountered with using this method is that he expected all of the adults in his life to engage in problem solving with him. That often didn't happen, particularly at school, where he was often silenced and told what to do. His inability to articulate his concerns often led to outbursts or inappropriate behavior, which could easily have been circumvented. It was very frustrating."

Carolyn's family's experiences with the local school district have been nothing short of horrific. (Not only did one of her children's schools "white out" a mandated accommodation on her child's IEP so that they wouldn't have to carry it out: the school reported her to child welfare for suspected child neglect. That investigation culminated with the child welfare investigator declaring the investigation a complete waste of time—and blaming Carolyn for the fact that it occurred!) What has allowed her to keep going— to keep advocating on her children's behalf under often painful and humiliating circumstances—is the support of her child's occupational therapist, someone who both understands the severity of her child's struggle and who remains optimistic that change is possible: "Having the support of the OT was great—knowing I wasn't making this up (that there *was* something wrong) and that there were things we could do about it."

Eve's family ended up giving up on the public school system entirely, something that added to the family's stress by layering on massive financial pressures as well. "We eventually pulled our child from public school and put her in a private school we couldn't afford (which meant that we had to live off our credit cards and go deeply into debt), all because she had no one at the school who believed in her and who didn't shame her, and because she was so different, she became a target and was bullied by other kids regularly. I wish I had found some kind of an education advocate who could have walked me through the process of requesting help and documenting my efforts, and I wish I had attempted to get the school district to pay for her private school since they weren't able to meet her needs. But I don't honestly know if any of that would have been possible. She now goes to a private school for kids with learning disabilities, and a lot of the kids there are quirky, with various learning disabilities and mental health issues. There, she fits in, and she is taught by a staff of people who believe in her and who understand and aren't offended by her behaviors. The classes are very small, and this helps her teachers to be receptive to her needs, but that also makes the school very expensive."

So what can schools do to make things better for families like Carolyn's and Eve's?

They can ensure that all staff members receive adequate training in supporting all students with mental health challenges, as well as their families, and by ensuring that these issues are adequately addressed in the school curriculum (to create an environment of support and understanding within the entire school community).

These kinds of seismic shifts in thinking take time—and schools can't fight these battles on their own.

"Teachers need our help," says Darcy Gruttadaro, director of the NAMI Child and Adolescent Action Center, in Arlington, Virginia. "They go into the field of education because they want to do right by kids." And doing right by kids, circa 2016, means looking out for the early warning signs that a child is struggling so that children who would benefit from additional supports can be referred for diagnosis and treatment right away. It's in the best interest of the school to do this (fewer discipline problems for teachers and principals), and it's in the best interests of children and families to do this (children respond better to treatment when that treatment starts sooner rather than later). And, of course, we also need the necessary community supports to make this kind of early intervention possible, a topic we'll be returning to in Chapter 14 when we talk about wraparound care and other supports for children—and families—who are struggling.

## Discipline Revisited

If your child's school days prediagnosis were characterized by trips to the principal's office, phone calls home, and suspensions for behavioral issues, you may be wondering how having a diagnosis and an IEP in place will change things on the discipline front.

Most families find that things improve significantly, that the school becomes more willing to work with the child and the family to resolve behavioral issues in the classroom, as opposed to immediately resorting to suspensions.

"From a school perspective, obtaining a diagnosis gave the school a better understanding of [Skyler's] illness, but it also forced them to perceive his behavior differently," explains Leigh. "They could no longer just dismiss it and mete out consequences. That had been their go-to strategy in the past. Once we had a diagnosis and an IEP, they were forced to reconsider his illness as a disability that required certain approaches, resources, and tools. It wasn't perfect, but it was better than suspensions, which had him feeling like a failure and a loser."

Of course, many behavioral problems can be avoided if an adult stops to consider the child's needs (there is logic behind every behavior) and then works with the child to find ways of getting those needs met in ways other than resorting to inappropriate behavior. This approach is significantly different from relying on rewards and punishments—strategies that often trigger more disruptive behavior.

"A common misperception when dealing with disruptive behavior is that we just have not found a strong enough motivator for students to behave," says Leah M. Kuypers in *The Zones of Regulation: A Curriculum Designed to Foster Self-Regulation and Emotional Control*. "However, students do not act out because of a lack of motivation for a reward. . . . Students often act out because they don't know how to make better choices. Students need to be taught what they could do differently and be given the opportunities to practice the skills in a safe and supportive environment."

Susan E. Craig makes a similar point in *Reaching and Teaching Children Who Hurt: Strategies for Your Classroom*. "Using consequences to achieve compliance with school or classroom rules is seldom effective, and may, in fact, escalate negative behaviors when children are unable to comply for reasons neither they nor their teacher understand."

It makes more sense to take a problem-solving approach with students who are feeling frustrated or anxious than one that is purely punitive, says Craig. "Teach children how to think out loud about the resources they can use to solve a problem or reach a goal." It's also important to head off problems by providing students with clear explanations of what is expected of them, providing them with additional support during activities or at times of the day that are particularly difficult for them ("This helps to avoid power struggles and lets a child who is experiencing difficulty know you are on his or her side"), offering them opportunities to make choices about how they spend their time, and providing them with opportunities to collaborate with the teacher to find solutions when they are feeling stuck.

Don't overlook the role of sensory supports as a means of avoiding potential discipline problems in the classroom. "If the student's sensory needs aren't being accommodated, the student will still find a way to meet his or her sensory needs, but in a more disruptive and maladaptive manner," explains Kuypers in *The Zones of Regulation*. "Some students find it effective to use sensory supports at their seats that help their need to touch things (such as playing with a fidget ball), move (such as sitting on a therapy ball rather than a chair), and work their muscles (such as tying a stretch band or fabric around the legs of a desk so the children can pull and push against it with [their] legs). Other students require more intense activities, such as heavy work, running, climbing, crashing, swinging, and burrowing under pillows/bean bags, to help them reach an optimal state of alertness for learning and socializing."

Finally, it's critically important that students receive the message that the teacher (like their parent) is on their side: "When teachers are judging them, students will sabotage the teacher by not trying," writes Carol S. Dweck in *Mindset: The New Psychology of Success*. "But when students understand that school is for them—a way for them to grow their minds—they do not insist on sabotaging themselves."

## When Is Home Schooling the Best Option?

If attending classes in a traditional classroom setting isn't working out well for your child, you may need to consider other options: perhaps a modified classroom setting or a switch to a different school. Some families find that none of these options are tenable (either because of a lack of viable options in their community, because school-based learning isn't a good fit for their child, and/or because they can't afford to pay hefty private school fees), in which case home schooling becomes the best possible option, either by choice or by default.

Ruby knew she had to consider home schooling when kindergarten proved to be a disaster for her twins, with both exhibiting extreme school anxiety. "My son was vomiting on the way to school and peeing constantly. Everyone in kindergarten sends a change of clothes. I was sending four and five changes of clothes every day," she recalls. Despite her best efforts to work with the school ("I was in there every day. I basically went to kindergarten"), it was impossible to make school work for her kids. "We're home-schooling now, and everybody's a lot happier."

Priya remembers having a lightbulb moment—a moment when it became clear to her that school was no longer an option for her son Ravi, who has been diagnosed with Asperger syndrome. It occurred in the wake of an incident when Ravi, after 3 years of misery, refused to step foot inside the school. Home schooling wasn't something she had wanted, but she felt that it had become the last, best option for Ravi, who was both frustrated by and terrified of school. "We never wanted to home school. I had always believed, 'Kids need to go to school.' But then we realized, this kid *can't* go to school. He just can't do it.' And so we decided to pull him out. We told him: 'You know what? You don't have to go back there. Let's do school at home.'" And that changed everything for Ravi and for them. What Ravi needed was to have the source of his anxiety removed—and the source of that anxiety was school. After a period of completely unstructured learning ("For about 6 months he would completely reject any school-like activity," she recalls), Ravi's love of learning was rekindled. And a couple of years later, he made the decision on his own to go back to school—and he's never looked back: "He went back to school in middle school and he has been thriving and happy ever since."

## To High School . . . and Beyond

Many students take longer than 4 years to obtain all of their high school credits—and not just students who are experiencing mental health or development challenges. If your child is finding it difficult to cope with a full course load, taking fewer courses or limiting the number of homework-heavy courses that are taken at the same time can make the high school workload more manageable. And if your child is going through a particularly difficult time, taking a semester off to focus on getting better is time well spent. Education is not a race. It's okay if your child ends up taking a little longer to graduate, especially if it means experiencing better mental health along the way.

Michelle wonders about the appropriateness of the high school experience for certain students. "Martin [who has been diagnosed with generalized anxiety disorder] is now going through what John [who was diagnosed with depression with suicidal thoughts] did: a late high school diagnosis, failing 12th grade, self-esteem crisis, poor understanding on the part of the school. I wonder how we can structure education to serve these kids. I wonder if sending them to this big, bureaucratic place full of stress and competition and negativity contributed to their disease."

While the situation in each individual school and school district may be unique, all schools—public and private—are subject to legislation that governs students who are struggling with mental health issues. You will find it easier to advocate effectively on your child's behalf if you understand the specific policies and procedures in place in your jurisdiction. To learn how the educational system works and what types of in-school supports and accommodations may be possible, visit the education section of federal, state, and county government websites as well as the websites of education consultants, education attorneys, and nonprofit groups working in the area of education law and advocacy. Then make contact with parent support groups in your community (like your local chapter of NAMI) to obtain nitty-gritty advice on making the system work for your child.

Something else you'll want to start thinking about during your child's high school years is life after high school. If your child has an IEP in place, the school will help to guide you through the process of considering his postsecondary next steps. The IDEA recommends that such transition planning begin by the time a young person reaches 16 years of age—and even sooner if the need for earlier planning is noted in the IEP. Under the provisions of the IDEA, students must be invited to participate in any meeting that is focused on their postsecondary goals, whether those goals include postsecondary education, vocational training, employment, independent living, and/or community participation. According to the Bazelon Center for Mental Health Law, the goal is to come up with a coordinated (across agencies) results-oriented transition plan that spells out the student's own goals for himself and that takes into account his preferences, interests, needs, and strengths (PINS).

If your child has plans to continue his education at the postsecondary level, the two of you have some important decisions to make—namely, when he should head off to college and where.

### Assessing Your Child's Readiness for College

Some kids need a little more time to learn and grow before they are ready to leave home. That's okay. "Your child has to be stable before going to college," says young adult mental health advocate and lawyer Nancy L. Wolf of the educational consulting firm Your Bridge Forward. "Sometimes it makes sense to step back and say, 'Let's take a gap year' if your child isn't ready to head to college right away."

Resist the temptation to try to convince yourself that things will miraculously improve when your child heads off to college, she advises. Instead, recognize that the transition to college can be difficult for any student—and the process can be even tougher for a child who is struggling with an existing mental health, neurodevelopmental, and/or behavioral challenge.

It's important to keep your expectations realistic about what is possible for your child right now—and to not be too disappointed if it takes your child more than one try to make the transition from high school to college or if alternatives to a full-time residential college experience would work better for him. (Maybe he could commute to college while continuing to live at home or ease into his studies on a part-time basis.)

You'll also want to encourage your child to cut himself some slack in terms of setting expectations for himself: "We told him, 'Going to college in any way for you is successful,'" says Rashida, whose son, Elijah, who has been diagnosed with bipolar disorder and is commuting to college this year after a difficult experience living on campus last year. "'You have struggles that not everybody has.'"

### Choosing a Mental-Health-Friendly College

If your child has a preexisting mental health challenge, you will probably want to look for a mental-health-friendly college (a college that makes mental health services and supports a priority on campus), says Wolf.

So how do you go about finding a mental-health-friendly college?

For starters, don't assume that sky-high tuition bills guarantee your child the necessary supports. "The fact that a college has elite facilities is no guarantee that they pour that money into their mental health services," says Wolf. Instead of relying on a school's name, do a bit of digging to find out how well the college you're considering measures up on the mental health front. Find out if it has been recognized by the Jed Foundation (*jedfoundation.org*) for the quality of its mental health services. This non-profit has developed the mental health world equivalent of a *Good Housekeeping* seal of approval (JedCampus Seals) to recognize colleges with comprehensive mental health and suicide prevention programs.

You'll also want to look for the presence of peer-led support and advocacy groups like Active Minds or NAMI on Campus as well as comprehensive mental health services on campus (as opposed to students having to go to an off-campus clinic and/or find their own mental health services provider in town).

And you'll want to consider what types of supports might be available to your child via the school's disability rights office. (Tip: If your child needs a little extra support and you have the financial resources to pay for it, consider a school that offers additional services that aren't standard offerings at most schools: assistance with social skills and independent living skills, for example.)

And, speaking of disability rights, you'll want to look for a school that has a reputation for honoring the provisions of the ADA. According to the Bazelon Center for Mental Health Law, far too many colleges respond to mental health issues on campus in ways that violate the provisions of this key piece of legislation: "Under the ADA, colleges and universities may not exclude students because of their mental health needs, except when the student cannot meet academic and behavioral standards even with treatment and other help. In addition, schools must provide students with disabilities 'reasonable accommodations'—modifications to normal rules and procedures that enable students to continue and succeed in higher education."

Which raises the question—what happens if a student needs to take a break from her studies for mental health reasons? How does the school handle requests for mental health leave (as opposed to requests for physical health leave)? According to Wolf, some colleges require students returning after mental health leave to reapply and to submit medical documentation demonstrating that they are stable—whereas "If you break your leg, they don't require that you submit a doctor's note saying that your leg has healed." And yet the law is pretty clear on this front: "The person has to be a direct threat to himself or others" for the college to refuse to allow the student to return to campus after a mental health crisis. Sadly, as you'll discover as you conduct your research, there's a major gap between what colleges should be doing and what they're actually doing to meet the mental health needs of students on campus. (More about this in Chapter 14.)

### Offering Support during the College Years

Your relationship with your child is changing. He's heading off to college. But that doesn't mean he no longer needs your support.

"Parents still have an integral role to play in their students' lives," explains Alison Malmon, executive director and founder, Active Minds, Inc. "By showing them that you love them and you support them no matter what they're going through or who they are, you can be that safe space for them to return to."

You'll also want to be sure that your college-age son or daughter knows how to tap into additional services and supports, both on and off campus. Start with on-campus supports because it's a lot less overwhelming to try to access those supports when you're in crisis than it is to try to find a provider who is covered by your insurance. There are also all kinds of other mental health apps, online forums, national suicide prevention hotlines, and crisis text supports that "everyone can have at their fingertips and access 24/7," notes Malmon. She recommends that parents ensure that students know about the following national crisis support resources so that they can reach help whenever they need it:

- National Suicide Prevention Lifeline: 1-800-273-TALK.
- National Crisis Text Line: Text the word START to 741-741 (you don't get charged the texting fees and it will not show up on a bill).

And, of course, you'll want to have a conversation about the importance of reaching out for support when you're struggling—a strategy that may seem intuitive to you, as a parent, but that might not be quite so obvious to a young person. According to Active Minds, young adults between the ages of 18 and 24 are far less likely to reach out for help than older adults. That's why it's so important for young people to hear this message, says Malmon: "If you're struggling—if you're not feeling like yourself—if life isn't what you want it to be, talk to somebody about it. It could be a counselor, it could be a friend, it could be a parent. And know that you're not alone. There are a lot of people who love you. And seeking help is a sign of strength."

Students who are heading off to college with an existing diagnosis benefit from an additional pep talk—one that encourages them to learn and grow in the wake of that diagnosis. "Help students recognize that their mental health diagnosis is not their life story," says Malmon. "Students need to hear 'Maybe you have a diagnosis of depression or maybe you have struggled with an eating disorder, but you are a person above and beyond that disorder and that struggle—and the purpose of this next phase of life is to continue to learn who you are.'" A student's existing diagnosis is not going to go away—and this is a time to learn how to manage that diagnosis in a new environment—but, at the same time, "it's a great time to learn more about those other facets of yourself in a way that you might not have been able to do when you were in high school or grade school."

In other words, it's about daring to imagine the best possible life for yourself.

More on this theme in Chapter 13.

# 11

# The Friendship Department

Friendships can be difficult for children who are struggling with mental health challenges. Depending on the nature of their difficulties, they may have a hard time initiating or maintaining friendships.

"Gabriel has always struggled to make friends," says his mother, Laura. Gabriel has been diagnosed with Asperger syndrome and is currently being assessed for OCD. "He is extremely earnest, and so he isn't very popular with other kids."

"Friendships are hard for Madalyn," adds Rebecca, whose daughter has been diagnosed with learning disabilities. "She can be volatile and unpredictable. This past year, she was in a different classroom from the majority of her peers, and she wasn't sure how to enter into play with them when they did have the opportunity to play at recess."

> Aiden has a horrible time making friends and maintaining friendships. It crushes him. It is horrible to watch, and it breaks my heart.
> —Tara, mother of Aiden, who has been diagnosed with autism and ODD

Fortunately, there are things you can do to help your child learn how to make and keep friends. These skills don't come easily or naturally to all children, after all. And helping your child improve her social skills will reduce her vulnerability to being bullied—a significant problem for many children with mental health or development issues and a situation that can increase the severity of mental health challenges in a child who is already struggling. In addition to helping your child work on learning how to regulate his emotions and his attention (two skills that lay the groundwork for success on the relationship front), you'll want to give him opportunities to learn the art and science of being a friend.

## Helping Your Child Learn How to Make and Keep Friends

"Gabriel and I have always had a very honest relationship about his issues. From the time he was very young, I explained to him that his brain worked differently and that's why he had an educational assistant or a laptop at school—or why he had trouble figuring out what other kids were thinking," says Laura. "We still have these conversations, where we dissect a social encounter to see what may have gone wrong. This takes time, though, and these conversations don't always happen at the most convenient time. We'll even role-play what to do next time. This has often been helpful for him, and it highlights for me how much he wants to do better."

The approach that Laura has chosen to take with her son—helping Gabriel figure out the unwritten rules of social engagement by analyzing social encounters that haven't worked out very well for him, while providing him with the opportunity to role-play different outcomes—is one of the most practical and effective things a parent can do to help a child work on his social skills. The examples are relevant to the child (because they're drawn from his real-world experience), and he has a vested interest in finding alternative solutions (because he's already seen what can happen when the situation isn't handled as well as it could be). Laura can also help Gabriel generalize (or carry over) his learning to other, similar situations, so that he doesn't have to spend quite so much time studying at the School of Hard Knocks.

Laura can also allow fictional characters to step in for the people Gabriel might encounter in the real world by discussing the experiences of different characters in movies or books that she and Gabriel share. Susan E. Craig, author of *Reaching and Teaching Children Who Hurt: Strategies for Your Classroom*, suggests asking children what they think a minor character in a book or movie is thinking or feeling so that they are encouraged to adopt a perspective other than that of the main character. This gives children practice in switching perspectives—a difficult skill for many children to master.

Here's another exercise suggested by Craig that works on the same skill set: have your child describe the view from various points in the same room. This will help her see that there are many different ways of looking at the same situation.

Another important lesson for kids to learn is that conflict in relationships is normal and that relationships can be repaired. The best way to teach this lesson, of course, is to live it. Let your child see that while the two of you don't always agree about everything (and sometimes you may even disagree rather heatedly), the relationship endures because you do the hard work required to fix things when something's broken. You say sorry for being grumpy about something that really didn't matter. You let the other person know that the relationship is important to you. You learn from your mistakes. You move on.

If your child has entered the teen years, you may find that she's a bit more reluctant to talk about her friendship struggles, perhaps because of her emerging sense of privacy, or because she's embarrassed that she's having difficulty on this front. You can keep the conversation going by letting your child know you are always willing to talk about anything that is worrying her and by expressing optimism that things will get better as her relationship skills improve. You can also help her identify any behaviors that might be making things more difficult for her on the friendship front (not looking people in the eye when she is speaking to them, speaking too quietly or too loudly, or interrupting other people repeatedly, for example) and provide her with opportunities to practice more effective behaviors (making eye contact, speaking at a more appropriate volume, or remembering that a conversation involves listening as well as speaking). You can encourage her to become a social skills detective by looking for opportunities to watch more friendship-savvy peers in action, so she can pick up tips on interacting more easily and naturally with peers and apply her observations to future social situations.

What more can you do to help a child who is struggling on the friendship front?

### Start Out by Considering What Is Realistic for Your Child Right Now

Not all children are social butterflies, and not all children have had a chance to develop the underlying skills that allow friendships to thrive. It's important to respect your child's temperament and to acknowledge where he is developmentally as you look for ways to encourage your child to continue to work on his friendship skills. You might find that it works well to encourage your child or teenager to participate in extracurricular activities (he is bound to have at least one interest in common with people he meets while participating in a particular activity) or to invite a friend to join him for a family activity that is likely to be particularly appealing to the other child (a trip to the amusement park, a baseball game, or a favorite restaurant, for example). It's best to start out by inviting one friend along (inviting two friends could lead to your child being left out) and by keeping initial outings brief (so that your child can handle the friendship demands, and the friend has such a positive experience that he wants to come back again).

## Get to Know the Parents of the Other Children in Your Child's Class

You may not necessarily score any birthday party invitations on your child's behalf if the children aren't friends, but the other parents are more likely to have something positive to say about your child (or even to help reframe your child's behavior so that it makes sense to their children) if they have an existing relationship with you.

## Team Up with Your Child's Teacher

Have a conversation with your child's teacher about your child's efforts on the friendship front. Your child's teacher may be able to come up with practical strategies for helping your child foster friendships and work on his social skills. With younger children, for example, the teacher could pair your child up with a compatible classmate for classroom projects, and provide opportunities for your child to shine socially by sharing a special hobby or talent with his peers.

Jodi—whose son, Kyle, has been diagnosed with Asperger syndrome, a learning disability, generalized anxiety disorder, and ADHD—feels that schools have an important role to play in supporting friendships. She explains: "My son made a good friend in third grade, but the school messed up and decided not to put him with the friend in fourth grade. They remained friends over a period of time, but ultimately theirs did not become a lasting friendship. The school did the same thing between fourth grade and fifth grade. Parents need to insist that if their child has a friend—even if it's just one—the school needs to make sure that the children are kept together year after year." Of course, it's important to recognize that the school has to factor in the needs of both children and that your child's teacher may have a different perspective than you do on the pros and cons of keeping the two friends in the same class. What you want to do is spark a dialogue with the school so that these issues can be consciously considered and an appropriate decision can be reached.

## Help Your Child to Understand the Mechanics of Relationship Repair

Things go wrong in friendships. When human beings are involved, it's not a matter of if but when. Help your child understand how to go about dealing with an angry outburst or miscommunication that is threatening to derail a friendship, as opposed to simply feeling bad about what happened (which doesn't do anything to solve the problem and increases the odds of a child becoming anxious or depressed because he is upset about the relationship breakdown). Help your child brainstorm possible solutions (apologize for the angry outburst or have a conversation to clear up the miscommunication) and practice acting on these solutions through role playing.

### Get Creative When It Comes to Troubleshooting Specific Friendship Challenges

When Susan's son Jacob was forced to take some time off from school to deal with his anxiety problems, she noticed that he was becoming increasingly isolated from his peers. That spurred her to take action. "My son was definitely lonely," she recalls. "Being fifteen and boys, his friends didn't know what to say to him or how to react to him. So, being boys, they just didn't contact him at all. They are also teenagers who are caught up in their own lives. They just don't stop to consider that another person might be lonely. We organized a few ball hockey games for a couple of his friends to come by and play. It was a relaxing, nonthreatening way to gather the teens together. There wasn't time for any huge conversations, so the teens didn't feel awkward. Adults were present, too, to help keep the conversation going."

### Work on Other Related Issues and Skills

Understand that friendship difficulties can be linked to difficulties with self-regulation and that improvements in the area of self-regulation will often lead to improvements on the friendship front as well. Christine found that her son Will's friendship difficulties didn't start to improve until after he began taking medication (for severe ADHD and an anxiety disorder). "Will went from being a popular, well-liked kid to being excluded from most birthday parties and playdates," she recalls. "He was very aware of this, and his self-esteem plummeted. I'm happy to say that Will had at least a few very good friends who continued to invite him over and who came to our house to play. Will worked through this by focusing on those friendships. He also started spending a lot more time with family, and we worked hard at building up his self-esteem. Will worked with a psychologist on expected and unexpected behaviors, as she thought this would help him control the impulsive behavior that was contributing to Will's social isolation. It didn't work, though. Will simply had no impulse control and very little ability to regulate his emotions. Since he began medication, his social skills have been improved and he's been able to make many new friends."

Kim has been able to identify a couple of factors that finally made things better for her son, Tom, who has been diagnosed with ADHD as well as a learning disability: "Tom had difficulty making friends and maintaining friendships during his primary school years, but he now has some very close friends. I think that maturity, growth in the area of his social skills, and a better understanding of the 'hidden curriculum' of friendships combined with medication has definitely helped Tom."

Mark says that what changed for his son, Dawson (who has been diagnosed with reactive attachment disorder, a moderate developmental disability, and an anxiety disorder) was finally finding the right group of friends: "Dawson's closest friends right now are other children who have similar difficulties. It seems that they can relate to and show empathy for one another and be far more understanding when one of them is having an off day."

Remind yourself that quality is more important than quantity when it comes to friendships. Your child doesn't need a lot of friends, but he will benefit from having at least one good friend. If you had a lot of friends when you were growing up, you may find it difficult to imagine that your child could be happy with so many fewer friends. That's part of the challenge of being a parent: recognizing that there are differences between you and your child and allowing him to come up with his own recipe for thriving in the world, even if that recipe is radically different from yours.

> Kyle was always the kid who never got invited to other kids' birthday parties, but he always invited them to his (and they did attend). I think the loneliness and friendship issues were something that we worried about more than he did. We know how important friends are, but he seemed to find other things to occupy himself. He was happy with his own company. Today, though, he has a great group of friends and is fairly social. I think kids have to want to have friends; parents can't push them to have friends.
>
> —Jodi, mother of Kyle, who has been diagnosed with Asperger syndrome, a learning disability, generalized anxiety disorder, and ADHD

## Why Your Child Is More Likely to Be Bullied

It's not your imagination: children with mental health challenges *are* more likely to be bullied than other children. A study published in 2009 in the journal *Child Development* found that children who show signs of depression, anxiety, or excessive aggression at the time they enter first grade are at risk of being chronically victimized by their classmates 2 years later. And a study published in 2006 in the medical journal *Pediatrics* concluded, "Some behaviors may evoke or reinforce aggressive encounters and possibly place some children in the position of being easy targets for bullies." This doesn't mean that it's right—that your child deserves to be bullied because she acts a certain way. What it means is that it's a reality: your child may be more vulnerable as a result of those behaviors.

The good news is that addressing children's challenges may help to reduce bullying, by giving kids the skills they need to navigate the complex world of elementary school social relationships. And some recent research highlights the fact that schools can make a very big difference in the lives of children who are struggling to master these all-important social skills by encouraging prosocial behavior in all of their students.

A study published in a 2012 issue of the open-access scientific journal *PLOS ONE* found that encouraging 9- to 11-year-olds to engage in acts of kindness toward others led to both increased happiness and increased popularity. The researchers explained the significance of this finding in terms of its potential to reduce bullying and increase student mental health: "Being well liked by classmates has ramifications not only for the individual, but also for the community at large. For example, well-liked preadolescents exhibit more inclusive behaviors and less externalizing behaviors (i.e., less bullying) as teens. Thus, encouraging prosocial activities may have ripple effects beyond increasing the happiness and popularity of the doers. Furthermore, classrooms with an even distribution of popularity (i.e., no favorite children and no marginalized children) show better average mental health than stratified classrooms, suggesting that entire classrooms practicing prosocial behavior may reap benefits, as the liking of all classmates soars."

## How Being Bullied Affects Mental Health

Approximately one in three children is bullied on an ongoing basis, putting them at risk for a wide range of mental and physical health problems throughout childhood and into adulthood. Children may be bullied for reasons related to appearance, social status, sexual orientation, race, religion, or because they are shyer and more introverted than other children. Regardless of what triggers the bullying, the fallout can be devastating.

According to a 2011 article reporting on the health impact of bullying during childhood, published in the *Journal of Pediatric Psychology*, "Early peer victimization has been associated with depression, anxiety, suicidal ideation, low self-esteem, and psychosomatic complaints, as well as increased externalizing problems, poor school performance, and higher rates of school avoidance. . . . Chronic stressors may weaken immune defenses and make individuals more vulnerable to illnesses, thus leading to the development of physical health problems."

An article in a 2006 issue of the medical journal *Pediatrics* noted: "Being the victim of a bully during the first years of schooling contributes to maladjustment in young children. Prevention and intervention programs aimed at reducing mental health problems during childhood should target bullying as an important risk factor. . . . Our findings suggest that bullying uniquely contributes to symptoms of maladjustment among young children and that bullying has harmful consequences for the victims, whether or not they also bully others."

Bullying can also be a problem during the teen years, with boys being more likely to experience acts of physical bullying (being hit or punched) and girls being more likely to experience relational aggression (being subject to gossip, being excluded from groups, and other hurtful activities designed to leave them feeling isolated and alone). Teenagers who are subjected to bullying behavior—either face-to-face or electronically via private message, online post, or in chat rooms—are likely to feel stressed, anxious, and afraid. Some may even consider ending their lives. A 2007 study found that teenagers who were bullied at school on a regular basis were five times as likely to have experienced suicidal thoughts and four times as likely to have attempted suicide as students who had not been bullied.

Because teenagers are less likely than younger children to confide in parents about experiences involving bullying, it is more important than ever to be alert to any signs that your child is being bullied. You should consider the possibility that your teenager is being bullied if you notice physical changes (unexplained cuts and bruises, missing or damaged clothing and other items) and changes in your teen's behavior (difficulty sleeping, eating more or less than usual, a lack of interest in activities she normally enjoys, complaints about headaches or stomachaches). In such a situation, it is important to raise your concerns with your teenager and to reassure her that you will help her deal with the problem. Then follow through as soon as possible, by soliciting the support of other caring adults in your child's life, perhaps a teacher who can act as a confidant at school or a favorite aunt who can offer a much-needed diversion and tons of TLC. Your teenager is counting on you.

## Why Your Child May Bully Others

Of course, there's another piece of the bullying puzzle to be considered: why some children with mental health problems end up bullying others.

A group of researchers decided to tease out the answer to this question by conducting a series of studies looking at peer rejection and the development of aggressive behavior problems in children. They wanted to find out whether antisocial behavior increases as a result of experiencing the stress of being rejected by other children or whether some other mechanism was at work. The researchers concluded that what was really going on was that, in the aftermath of being rejected by their peers, these children missed out on the opportunity to socialize with other children and, as a result, they fell behind their peers in terms of figuring out how social relationships work. More specifically, because they weren't playing with other children on a regular basis, they weren't mastering the same skills that their peers had the opportunity to master—skills like "cooperation, empathy, perspective taking, intention-cue detection, social problem solving, and response evaluation that inhibit aggressive behaviors." As a result, it was likely that the rejected child was more aggressive than his peers due to "lack of exposure to positive peer-group influences that inhibit aggressive behavior rather than [an] . . . exacerbation of antisocial tendencies," the researchers reported in a 2003 issue of the journal *Child Development*.

## What You Can Do to Reduce the Chance That Your Child Will Become a Victim or a Bully

Up until now we've been focusing on the fallout of bullying. Now let's shift gears and talk about what parents can do to reduce the likelihood that their child will experience (or engage in) bullying problems in the first place.

### *Treat Mental Health Problems Early*

If you suspect that your child is dealing with a mental health challenge, seek a diagnosis and treatment early. Information is power: knowing what you are dealing with allows you to help your child to develop the types of skills that will reduce his vulnerability to bullying. And spread the word about the importance of universal early-childhood mental health assessments so that bullying can be stopped before it starts. In a 2003 article published in the *Journal of Applied School Psychology*, researchers recommended early and regular screening for anxiety, withdrawal, and stress-induced illnesses so that children can be identified and school personnel and parents can intervene to reduce the likelihood of bullying. "Low levels of aggression and anxiety may be the most effective protective factors," they wrote.

## Work on Your Child's Emotional Literacy and Social Skills

If you are waiting for a diagnosis or for treatment to begin, there's a lot you can do in the meantime. See the discussion of emotional literacy in Chapter 7 and see the book website (*www.anndouglas.net*) for some suggested resources.

## Teach Your Child to Ask for Help

The research has noted that children who have been bullied need to be taught how to ask for help in a way that strengthens relationships, minimizes conflict, and encourages the other person to want to help. And they can ask for help to engage in positive conflict resolution, which will reduce their risk of being bullied again. "Education regarding the ineffectiveness of strategies such as aggression is also important," the researchers stress, as is putting in place programs designed to foster supportive social networks at school (for example, support circles and mentoring programs).

## Be Prepared to Advocate on Your Child's Behalf

Take your child's concerns seriously and help her come up with a plan for dealing with bullying. Don't be afraid to reach out to teachers, coaches, school administrators, and other parents for support in dealing with the bullying problem and coming up with solutions that will work for your child.

## Help Your Child Develop Strong Relationships

Once again, it all comes down to relationships. As bullying expert and psychologist Debra Pepler likes to put it, "Bullying is a relationship problem that requires relationship solutions." In addition to encouraging strong relationships within the family, you'll want to encourage your child to develop the following relationships.

• *A strong relationship with a teacher.* Children who face a higher risk of engaging in bullying or being bullied are less likely to become bullies or victims if they have a warm and affectionate relationship with their teacher. That's the key finding to emerge from a university study of Canadian first graders. The researchers concluded that children's relationships with teachers, like their relationships with their peers, play a critical role in shaping their social-behavioral development.

- *A strong relationship with a peer.* Having one good friend may be all that is needed to protect a child from being bullied. Says Laura, "A really popular boy at school—with a very kind heart—has taken a liking to Gabriel and is very kind to him. They aren't friends per se, but they are friendly, and this has gone a long way toward giving Gabriel credibility at school. Gabriel must be okay if Joel says so." Likewise, having a friend provides the child with the opportunity to acquire the very types of social skills that may protect the child from becoming a victim—or a bully—later on.

- *A strong relationship with you.* Your child needs to feel the strength of your caring and to know that you'll do what you can to make the situation better, starting right now.

It can be heartbreaking to watch a child who is already struggling being bullied, or to see him resort to bullying behaviors because his social skills are lagging behind those of his peers. I've been in both places as a mom, and it's hard to say which is worse: watching your child be bullied or be the bully.

Bullying may be prevalent, but that doesn't mean we should accept it as a childhood rite of passage. We need to take action to prevent our children from becoming victims of bullying in the first place (or engaging in bullying behaviors themselves); to support them in dealing with any bullying issues that arise; to help our kids develop the social and attention regulation skills that allow friendships to thrive; and to work with other adults to create caring communities that are characterized by kindness and mutual respect. And, of course, we need to be our children's role models on this front, modeling, in our dealings with other people, the type of prosocial behaviors we hope they will exhibit. We have to be prepared to walk the talk.

# 12

# Finding Community

You are not alone. That's the most important thing to know when you are caring for a child with mental health challenges. Other parents understand because they are walking this path too, and they can lighten your load and decrease your learning curve by sharing what they've learned along the way.

In this chapter, we'll be talking about finding community—a community that can be a source of support and information to you as you try to make sense of the journey you find yourself on, and a community that can provide you with the strength and resources you need to advocate effectively for your child. As Kristin Neff notes in her book *Self-Compassion: Stop Beating Yourself Up and Leave Insecurity Behind*, "Feelings of connectedness, like feelings of kindness, activate the brain's attachment system. . . . People who feel connected to others are not as frightened by difficult life circumstances and are more readily able to roll with the punches."

> Find a community—a village— of people, whether in person or online, and be honest about your struggles.
> —Rebecca, mother of Madalyn, who has been diagnosed with learning disabilities and is awaiting a mental health diagnosis

## Seeking Support

There are few things in life more powerful or affirming than having a heart-to-heart conversation with someone who truly understands what you're going through because of having walked a similar path. Such is the power of peer-to-peer support.

200

Sometimes this type of support happens naturally. You start talking with another parent and discover that you each have a child who has been struggling with the same types of challenges, and the conversation simply takes off from there. At other times, peer-to-peer support occurs within a more structured setting: via an online or face-to-face support group, for example. Wherever or however it happens, the impact of receiving such support can be life changing.

"Parents need to seek out support from anyone they can," says Jackie, whose two sons, David and John, have been diagnosed with psychosis. "It's a very dark, scary, and long journey, and it can be very lonely. You need to know that you are not alone."

Cheyenne, whose daughter, Keisha, has been diagnosed with ADHD and anxiety, agrees. "You have to find the right people [to support you] or you will not survive. And they're out there. There's a secret underground network—and you have no idea who's in the network."

"I received a great deal of support from not-for-profit organizations and by connecting with families who had gone through or were going through the same experience," adds Lydia, whose son Thomas struggles with suicidal thoughts. "They will help you see you can get to the other side—to see your child laugh again, to enjoy the simple pleasures of life again."

"I find support from other parents who have children struggling with ADHD," says Christine. "We meet very informally over coffee or lunch and just talk about everything we've been through and how things are now."

"Parenting groups are wonderful," says Claire, whose son Owen was diagnosed with bipolar disorder, a personality disorder, and extreme anxiety. "You will meet parents from all walks of life who are dealing with children with mental health issues. It is so important to know that you are not alone."

Ruby, mother of two children on the autism spectrum, agrees: "You don't have to reinvent the wheel. Connect with another parent who has already been through this and who can walk you through the process."

Lisa, whose daughter, Laura, is awaiting a diagnosis, has learned to seek support on multiple fronts: "I reach out to my friends and my support system," she says. "I can't do it alone. I've tried."

Whether you decide to seek out support via an online or face-to-face support group is largely a matter of personal preference and what is available to you in your community. Some parents like the convenience (you can give and receive support 24 hours a day) and the relative anonymity (you don't have to use your real name) of tapping into support online. Others prefer to focus their efforts on getting to know other parents in their own community—people who are trying to make sense of the same school and mental health care systems and trying to advocate for their children within them.

Ask your child's doctor and teachers as well as other parents for leads on such groups operating in your community. You might also want to make contact with NAMI (*www.nami.org*) and the National Federation of Families for Children's Mental Health (*www.ffcmh.org*). See the book website (*www.anndouglas.net*) for additional resources.

> When one of us tells the truth, he makes it easier for all of us to open our hearts to our pain and that of others.
>
> **—Mary Pipher**

**NOTE:** If you are planning to attend a medical conference to learn more about your child's illness, you may be able to claim your registration fees and travel expenses under medical expenses on your tax return. The conference must focus specifically on your child's medical condition (as opposed to general health and well-being). See IRS Publication 502 for details.

## Taking a Break

Sometimes you need another parent who has been in your shoes to remind you of the importance of taking a break. You may feel as if you can't take a break from your child when he's going through such a hard time. This is when it helps to have someone else tell you that you need to take a break—even a short break—to rejuvenate yourself so that you can continue to provide your child with the love and support he will need over the long term. You can't risk burning out. There's too much at stake for your child. And research has shown that when a caregiver experiences burnout, it is more difficult for the person who is struggling with a mental health challenge to stick with his treatment plan.

You also need to prevent burnout to allow yourself to be the type of parent you want to be. "When you are exhausted or not coping well yourself, you cannot deal with your child effectively," says Claire. "Being angry and exhausted will cause a barrier in your relationship. Take a break when you need to. And seek counseling and support."

"Take time for yourself to recharge. And give your family members the same," advises Mark, whose son, Dawson, has been diagnosed with reactive attachment disorder, a moderate developmental disability, and an anxiety disorder. "Use respite workers. Take a break or a timeout."

Respite care is a kind of glue that strengthens your family, providing you and your other children with a much-needed break from the responsibilities of caring for your child. It might involve in-home care (your child is cared for in your home while you spend time with other children and/

or catch up on household tasks, for example)—or out-of-home care (having your child receive residential respite care while you travel out of town to attend a family wedding, for example). In some cases, respite care is provided on a volunteer basis and/or subsidized by community agencies providing outreach support to families, but in most cases you will have to contract and pay for such support privately.

> **NOTE:** If your child is unable to dress, clean, or feed herself as a result of a physical or mental disability or requires constant supervision due to the nature of her illness, you may be able to claim the money you pay someone to come to your house to provide appropriate care as part of the Child or Dependent Tax Credit. (See IRS Publication 503 for details.) And if your child is "permanently and totally disabled" in the eyes of the IRS, you may qualify for the Earned Income Credit regardless of the age of your child—something that may help to free up funds to pay for much-needed respite care. (See IRS Publication 596.)

## Finding Allies at Work

Relationships at work can be strained by the fallout from a child's mental health, neurodevelopmental, or behavioral challenges. So, how do you reconcile your priorities and seek support from your work community?

It starts with acknowledging that work can be a major contributor to your stress and recognizing that adjustments might have to be made.

Some parents end up changing jobs or leaving the workforce entirely because it simply isn't possible to meet the needs of their child while upholding their responsibilities to their employer. "When I lost a well-paying but stressful job 3 years ago, I had to recognize that I couldn't balance life and work as long as I had my daughter's issues to manage," says Rebecca, mother of Madalyn. "So, I took a huge pay cut to work as an administrative assistant. The advantage is that I don't have to worry about my work life when I'm home. The disadvantage is that the reduced salary contributes to my stress."

"I ended up having to modify my work schedule so that I could drop Skyler off at school in the morning and pick him up after school, because I was afraid to have anyone else look after him," says his mother, Leigh. Skyler has been diagnosed with ADHD, anxiety, and depression. "It wasn't unusual for me to be called during the day to pick him up or to have to stay home when I realized that he wasn't in a good place emotionally to be at school."

Even if a parent's work schedule is relatively flexible, parents still need to make changes to meet their child's needs and their work commitments.

The resulting round-the-clock juggling act can send stress levels soaring sky-high.

"I work in a career where the demands of my personal life can largely be accommodated," says Mary, mother of Janine, who has a mild intellectual disability and is on the autism spectrum, and Fiona, who has been diagnosed with bipolar disorder. "I currently have to work from home quite frequently to enable me to get to Fiona's appointments. The trade-off is I regularly work on weekends to catch up. It is very difficult and draining. It also means there are interesting work projects and professional associations that I cannot get involved with because I have no time to give."

"I am self-employed and ended up having to put a lot of work aside and to hire someone else to help out so that I would have time to deal with all the appointments my daughter requires," says Sandra, mother of Sophie, who was diagnosed with moderate autism with global developmental delays. "It is not ideal, but I keep hoping that I will have time to catch up eventually. I get the basics done for now and catch up on administrative work as I can."

"I am lucky that I have a very understanding workplace that allows me great flexibility to take Adam to medical appointments, pick him up from school when he is sent home for aggressive behavior, and take care of any other needs that I must attend to," says his mother, Tami. "The flip side of this equation, however, is that I still have to get all my work done in a timely manner, which means having to find pockets of time during evenings and weekends, adding to my already high stress levels. I only wish my husband's employer was equally enlightened. It has been a recurring point of contention that we both work full-time and yet, because I have more flexibility in my job, I have taken on the majority of commitments related to Adam's ADHD."

Here are some tips that will help you deal with work–family conflict.

### Communicate Openly but Nonapologetically with Your Employer and Coworkers

You have nothing to apologize for, after all. Most people will end up dealing with some sort of family-related emergency at some point during their working lives. When their time comes, your coworkers will be seeking the very same types of workplace accommodations that you are seeking right now. Practice asking for the help you need in an open and unapologetic way until this becomes your default mode of response, for example: "My daughter is not well right now and we are going through some assessments. This is likely to require additional medical appointments, and she may not cope well at school. We are hoping for the best, but I need to talk to you about the times I need to be there—how to make that work with my job, which is also very important to me."

## Offer Solutions

Let your coworkers know what you intend to do to stay on top of your work-related commitments (or to what extent you will be able to keep on top of your work-related commitments right now) and let them know what support you need from them and for how long.

## Know Your Rights

Check in with the human resources department to find out how much family leave (both paid and unpaid) you are entitled to and talk to other people in your workplace who have faced similar challenges. They'll be able to give you the inside scoop on official (and unofficial) workplace accommodations that may be able to ease your stress level for now. And research your rights under the Family and Medical Leave Act (FMLA), which allows eligible employees of employers who are covered by the act to take unpaid, job-protected leave for up to 12 weeks in each 12-month period to care for a family member with "a serious health condition"—and which mandates that group health insurance coverage be continued for such employees "under the same terms and conditions as if the employee had not taken leave." (See the FMLA page of the Department of Labor website for more information: *www.dol.gov/whd/fmla*.)

It takes a village to raise a child—and you need to be prepared to call on your village to meet the needs of a child who is struggling. Connecting with other parents who are facing similar challenges, taking regular breaks from the demands of parenting, and finding allies at work will reduce your stress level and strengthen your capacity to love and support your child.

# Part V

# Recovery and Beyond

When you first started dealing with your child's challenges, it took everything you had just to get through the day. You didn't have anything left to invest in tomorrow. But now that you have been dealing with everything for a while, you may find yourself starting to think about the big picture—what the future may hold for your child. You may find yourself daring to dream again. That's what this next section of the book is all about.

In Chapter 13, we'll look at your hopes and dreams for your child and your family: what you hope your child will be able to achieve for herself and how your family intends to support those efforts. I'll be talking about what it means to recover as an individual and as a family and why it is important to distinguish between clinical recovery and personal recovery as your child and your family start to set recovery goals.

Then, in Chapter 14, we'll look at your hopes and dreams for a better mental health system for children and youth: what that system might be like and what you can do to help make it a reality. After all, working to improve the system for others is one way to find meaning in your family's struggle.

# 13

# Daring to Dream Again

The World Health Organization defines mental health as "a state of well-being in which the individual realizes his or her own abilities, can cope with the normal stresses of life, can work productively and fruitfully, and is able to make a contribution to his or her community."

The idea that it is possible for people who are living with mental illness to simultaneously strive for and experience positive mental health is at the heart of what is known as the recovery movement—an advocacy movement led by people living with mental health challenges.

> Realize that wellness is a constantly moving target. It looks different for every person at different times.
> —Shelley, whose daughter Alex has been diagnosed with depression

If your child has been diagnosed with a neurodevelopmental disorder (for example, an autism spectrum disorder), you may prefer the term *acceptance* to the term *recovery*, in recognition of the fact that your child's journey—and your journey as a family—is likely to involve both accepting the reality of the diagnosis and working to maximize your child's wellness and quality of life. Which term you prefer is largely a matter of semantics, but people in the autism community tend to have strong feelings about the word *recovery* (either strongly in favor or strongly against). Ultimately, you'll want to use the word that works best for you and that best describes your family's situation, whether that word is *recovery, acceptance,* or something else entirely.

It's also important to recognize that the journey toward recovery or acceptance—whatever you choose to call it—is a journey that your family is making, too, as you develop the capacity to thrive in new ways while simultaneously loving and supporting a family member who has a mental health, neurodevelopmental, or behavioral challenge.

## What Recovery Means

Envisioning recovery means moving beyond the kind of black-and-white thinking that characterizes people as being either healthy or ill by recognizing instead that a person can experience periods of wellness while living with a diagnosis. The idea that "personal recovery is possible even in the presence of current symptoms" is central to the concept of recovery, writes Mike Slade in his book *Personal Recovery and Mental Illness: A Guide for Mental Health Professionals*. This is because "clinical recovery is a subset of personal recovery."

By distinguishing between clinical recovery (medical recovery from illness) and personal recovery (learning to live a meaningful and hope-filled life despite the limitations of illness), people living with mental illness are able to find new purpose and meaning in their lives. They "come to view the mental illness experience as a bump in the road of their life, which they get over and move on from," according to Slade.

"Recovery is an extremely personal process," notes Rebecca Woolis in her book *When Someone You Love Has a Mental Illness: A Handbook for Families, Friends, and Caregivers*. "It is a journey that each person travels in his or her own way and time frame. It will be very subtle or gradual for some and more sudden or dramatic for others. This journey is not linear. It will inevitably take many twists, turns, and forward and backward movement. There may be times, especially in the beginning, when the person feels confused, discouraged, isolated, ineffective, and hopeless." What matters is that the person making this journey knows that others believe in him, have hope for his future, and will support him in achieving his dreams and goals.

So what does this mean to you as the parent of a child who has been diagnosed with a psychiatric disorder? It means . . .

### *Supporting Your Child in Adopting a Recovery Mindset*

You can do this by helping your child see her diagnosis as something that empowers rather than limits her. Her diagnosis can help her make sense of her experience, and she can use this information to make the best life and treatment choices for herself. "Love and encouragement is key," says Jackie, whose sons, David and John, have each been diagnosed with a psychotic disorder. "[The diagnosis] gives your child the best hope for staying on treatment, becoming stable, and eventually having independence and some sort of quality of life."

## Helping Your Child Envision Recovery

Try having conversations that focus on purpose, values, self-worth, and her ability to make a difference. Ask questions that encourage optimism and hopefulness and that encourage your child to anticipate the future and to dream. Share stories about individuals who overcame significant obstacles to go on to lead happy, fulfilling lives. And help your child identify opportunities to develop feelings of self-worth by helping others. "The challenge is to constantly help them find purpose every day, either school, work, or chores," says Jackie. "This helps with recovery because they start feeling confident again."

## Encouraging Your Child to Begin to Set Personal Recovery Goals

You want her to set goals that mesh with her hopes, dreams, and aspirations. Reading stories and watching movies about others who have overcome adversity can help to spark aspiration in a child who is having a difficult time envisioning anything beyond the status quo. Then help your child work toward achieving those goals.

You might be worried that your child will choose a goal she might not be able to achieve. According to Slade, this is better than not daring to have a goal at all: "The development of recovery goals which involve positive risk-taking may therefore, paradoxically, reduce harmful risk. They give someone a reason not to self-harm or self-neglect or be violent." Focusing on strengths creates possibilities while focusing on weaknesses leads to passivity. Emphasize what you want to nurture. As Slade puts it, "The more we seek out and elaborate actual and potential mental well-being, the less we see (and support and create) mental illness."

Just recognize that your child's goals for herself may be quite different from the goals you may have for her, notes Jennifer, whose daughter, Jessica, experiences physical and psychological problems related to tuberous sclerosis. She explains: "Though she has many challenges, Jess feels like she is an adult. Just because she doesn't have the cognitive capacity of other people her age doesn't mean she doesn't want the same things they do, like to go to the prom or to get married someday and have children of her own. But one of the most important things for me to realize is that independence doesn't look the same for Jessica as it does for me. I remember asking the therapist, 'When will I be able to leave her alone for 10 minutes to run to the grocery store?' and she just said, 'That's your goal, not Jessica's. That's not even on her radar.' That was so powerful. It's not my job to make her into what it would be convenient for me to make her into. It's my job to help her be the best Jessica she can be, and that means helping her reach her goals [for herself], not my goals for her."

### Helping Your Child Identify What Soothes Him and What Helps to Keep Him Well

That way, he can learn how to manage his illness and assume greater responsibility for his own care. You'll want to encourage him to:

- Consider medication, therapy, and other treatments as resources that can support his recovery.
- Spot and manage his personal triggers.
- Detect and manage symptoms of illness.
- Identify the most effective strategies for coping on a day-to-day basis.
- Develop a personal support network made up of friends and family.
- Understand the important role that lifestyle (sleep, exercise, nutrition, fun) plays in maintaining mental health.

This is another place where your record keeping will serve you and your child well. The downloadable forms at *www.guilford.com/douglas-forms* give you places to keep information about all of the above; refer to them along with your child if your child is having trouble recalling details.

If your child is still quite young—or he is quite impaired by illness—he may not be able to assume responsibility for making recovery decisions quite yet. That said, it's never too early to begin adopting a recovery mindset yourself and to start speaking the language of what is possible to your child.

## Emphasizing Love and Acceptance Is Key

"Your support and positive outlook will allow [your child] to thrive to the greatest extent possible," notes Woolis. Because the symptoms of mental illness tend to be cyclical, "you must be prepared to change with them" and be flexible in how you respond to your child's changing needs. You want to encourage your child to do as much as she can for herself while still feeling your love and support. You also want to provide the "steadying influence" of a calm, consistent, predictable, and structured environment by being clear about rules and expectations.

Acceptance provides similar opportunities for growth—for all family members. "Acceptance . . . liberates caregivers from the earlier burdensome belief that it is their duty to somehow solve the problem," writes David A. Karp in *The Burden of Sympathy: How Families Cope with Mental Illness*. "Once beyond their profound loss, some people come to a deep admiration and respect for their family members who bravely struggle with the unimaginable pain of mental illness. They no longer measure their loved one in terms of pre-illness potentials now gone. Their new aspiration is to help them to become as happy and productive as their [mental illness] will allow."

Andrew, whose son David has been diagnosed with schizophrenia, has learned to practice what he calls "radical acceptance." He explains: "Because David's schizophrenia has by its very nature impaired and limited the relationship we might have enjoyed with him over time, it has been hard to come to terms with what seems now like a mostly one-sided, almost utilitarian connection at times. Rarely, we seem to get something back that looks like affection or real care about us, but when we sense it, we notice and try to appreciate it for what it might be. We've had to work hard to accept our child for who he has become and not let our disappointment with the effects of the illness overshadow our ability to see and be grateful for the glimpses of his humanity and vulnerability. I think radical acceptance is called for, and parents need to aim for that while, at the same time, forgiving themselves if they fall short of that from time to time."

Alison also embraces the idea of acceptance. For her, acceptance is about empowerment—for her daughter Charlotte and herself. "I spent my whole life being embarrassed about my anxiety. I'm done with being embarrassed about it and my daughter's anxiety. People can think what they like."

For Danielle, whose daughter Jessie has been diagnosed with autism and anxiety, acceptance means unconditional love: "Sometimes you have to stop trying to 'fix' your kids and just be there for them."

## Celebrating Successes along the Way

Parenting a child with a mental illness is like running a marathon—except there is no finish line. So rather than holding out for a big celebration at some point in the future when everything will magically be perfect (!), doesn't it make a lot more sense to pause and celebrate anything that's celebration-worthy along the way?

It's a mind shift that works for parents like Mark, who is definitely in the mood to celebrate the progress that's been made by his son, Dawson (who has been diagnosed with reactive attachment disorder, moderate developmental delays, and an anxiety disorder). "I am not saying that this journey is over. I am saying that, for now, things are pretty great. For someone to go from being violently aggressive and manic several times a day to not becoming aggressive or having a meltdown in over a year is a gigantic feat on its own. But what's amazing about it is that Dawson is okay—not thrilled, but okay—with continuing with his trauma therapist. He loves his art therapy, and he is now working on social skills. He's also joined a local sports team. He is okay with the choices we have made and still loves us, so we must have done something right."

Andrew is also in a good place. "We feel guardedly optimistic. David is about to be discharged from [a psychiatric hospital] to live in a high-support home. We certainly have fears about the higher level of risk that comes with living in the community after 5 years in the institution. We don't know how well he will adjust or how well his needs will be met. We wonder how people on the street will react to him, given that he will obviously still be psychotic. We worry about his safety. We also worry about how he may inappropriately try to access our home, because this was a problem when he was on the streets, and this led to police involvement. We are more hopeful about some of the changes we've seen in him, but still unsure how much respect he'll have for our needs when he is able to travel to our home more easily. Our expectations overall are quite simple and basic: We hope he has a safe, clean home with decent food and social opportunities. We hope he has some recreational interests that bring him satisfaction. We hope he'll stay connected to our family to the extent that he can."

Laura is enthusiastic about the progress made by her son, Gabriel, who has been diagnosed with Asperger syndrome (now simply referred to as an autism spectrum disorder in DSM-5) and is currently being assessed for OCD. "What has been most surprising for me is how capable my son is. If you had told me before he was born about the challenges he would face, I would have been devastated. But he's turned out to be a good kid who is doing his best to be successful in life. It has been so satisfying seeing him succeed in high school. He's getting decent grades, making some friends, and getting involved. That has been lovely to see and something I couldn't have imagined when he was 3 or 4 years old."

Christine gets choked up talking about how far her son, Will, has come. Will has been diagnosed with severe ADHD and an anxiety disorder. "I love him beyond words. I'm also very proud of him. He had such a rough life at such an early age (prediagnosis), and I can't imagine the courage it took him to face each day. It brings me to tears just thinking about it."

Lydia, who has a number of children who struggle with mental illness, has learned to take each day as it comes. "My children are on what I call 'the other side' of their mental illness. They are shining bright right now. I know there may still be some rocky days in the future, but right now I am enjoying the peacefulness of where my family is, and that is what I will hold on to, and that is what will give me strength when the time comes [to deal with their challenges] again."

Cheyenne also feels that it's important to savor the gift of an extraordinary day—because that kind of day truly is a gift: "Days like today remind me that the laughing, smiling girl in the picture on my desk and in my memories is still here. I just don't always get to hang out with her because her illness takes over. The knowledge that days like this are possible and will happen in the future are the reason that I crawl out of bed on many days. Because there is a chance that each day could be that day."

Mary, mother of Janine, who has a mild intellectual disability and is on the autism spectrum, and Fiona, who has been diagnosed with bipolar disorder, can certainly relate to those feelings. "Our lives are a bit of a roller coaster. The good times are measured in moments and we make the most of them. Sometimes they are fleeting."

Her daughters have made significant progress and have achieved some hard-won victories—victories that she savors. "Janine is now 20. If you had asked me when she was 11 years old, I would have foreseen supportive living arrangements and social [security] as her only future. But the therapy, camps, activities, accommodations, tutoring, and love and support have paid off. She started reading at 17 years of age and has been able to attend a modified college program, make friends, and earn some money on her own. The future looks brighter at the moment. I think she can have a fulfilling life if she keeps on the path she is on.

"Fiona is a work in progress. She has just been through a particularly bleak period with lots of mood instability, impulsivity, anxiety, and irritability. She is with a new specialist and once more changing her medication. She is 2 years behind in high school and still has a long way to go to catch up. She also has no social life. She is a bright, loving, and creative person and I hope that as she matures things will improve. We take things day by day and appreciate each

> I'm learning, as my children head into adulthood, that the worry doesn't go away. John recently experienced the breakup of a long-term relationship. I was tempted to travel to him—a 6-hour trip—to make sure he was okay, but I checked my response as he seems to be coping. Still, knowing that he has had suicidal thoughts in the past, it is really, really hard not to worry.
>
> —Michelle, whose son, John, was diagnosed with depression with suicidal thoughts and whose other son, Martin, was diagnosed with generalized anxiety disorder

achievement. . . . The future is the great unknown. She wants to live independently someday. I hope we can get her there one small step at a time."

Giving herself permission to seize the moment is what is allowing Claire, whose son Owen has been diagnosed with bipolar disorder, a personality disorder, and extreme anxiety, to replenish herself after a period of burnout. "We have become more relaxed about day-to-day life. Our motto is 'one day at a time.' When we're having a great moment, we embrace it. The other day, my kids were not home. My husband and I put on a CD and danced in our living room. It was a stress-free moment and we had fun."

## Dealing with Setbacks

When a child is learning to walk, there are a lot of tumbles before he learns how to make his way across the room with ease. And yet many people are surprised or even disappointed when a person who is living with a mental illness encounters a setback.

They shouldn't be.

"Setbacks are normal and necessary in life—they are a sign of health, not illness," notes Slade in his book *Personal Recovery and Mental Illness*. It's how we respond to these setbacks that's important. Ideally, we want to respond with love and encouragement and treat these experiences as opportunities for learning, just as we did when our children were toddlers taking those wobbly first steps.

But, of course, we're only human, and so sometimes we find ourselves experiencing feelings of frustration. We don't want to watch our child lose his footing. We want to fast-forward to the part where our child is doing cartwheels and dancing around.

"The waxing and waning course of anxiety is a huge frustration," says Alison, mother of Charlotte. "Just as you think she's making progress, she starts to regress. I have to remind myself that it's really important to try to stay positive and keep moving forward, accepting that there will be setbacks."

What can you do to make the most of a setback, so that something positive comes out of the experience for your child?

> Stay in love with your children. Know in your heart that you haven't lost them. When they know that you are on their side, they will work 100 times more than any of us to come back. And when they return, they will be different. They will be stronger and know themselves in a completely new way.
> —Cat, mother of two teenagers who struggle with mental health challenges

*Help Your Child Identify the Early Warning Signs of a Setback*

These warning signs will be unique to each person living with a mental illness. You can help by discussing with your child any changes you've noticed in her behavior. You may have noticed changes to her eating or sleeping patterns, her social behavior, her mood, her energy level, or her communication patterns (impaired communications or the reappearance of delusions). Ask her how she is feeling, what patterns she has noticed in herself, and what steps she thinks she could take to try to avoid any further escalation in symptoms.

*Modify Any Environmental Factors That Might Make a Difference to Your Child's Difficulties*

These factors might be positive or negative and can include putting in place a healthy lifestyle plan (diet, exercise) and creating a safe and consistent home atmosphere.

*Have a Solid Crisis Plan in Place*

Get in touch with your child's doctor or therapist if the situation seems to warrant it. If in doubt, err on the side of caution. It's better to make one too many phone calls than one too few. (For more details on handling and planning for a crisis, see the following section of this chapter.)

*Take Setbacks in Stride*

Remind yourself of Mike Slade's take on setbacks: they're a sign of health, not illness. After all, your child can experience a setback only because he is moving forward, and if you stop to think about it, that's actually a pretty major positive, at least in the big picture. You'll also want to remind yourself how far you've traveled as a family—how much more wisdom and experience you have today than when you first headed out on this journey.

And if that journey has taken you to some unexpected places? "You also have to realize that your life is never going to look the way that you expected—and you just have to learn to embrace what is and be grateful for the blessings in the particular life you have," says Cheyenne. "But don't beat yourself up if you're not there yet—if your child is in crisis, you can't even think that way." So let yourself be wherever you are and don't feel guilty: "You're doing the absolute best that you can at that point with what you've been given, and that's all you can do."

## Handling a Crisis

Sometimes the word *setback* simply isn't up to describing what it is your family is experiencing. What you're experiencing is more like a full-blown crisis.

Claire, mother of Owen, recalls a recent crisis that had far-reaching implications for her family: "Our son was self-medicating his mental health issues with drugs and alcohol. He was not staying on his prescribed medication. He was getting into trouble with the law. All of this was devastating for us. And he was also devastated by what he had done—so devastated that he turned himself in to the police.

"Not only is this kind of experience devastating; it is humiliating and embarrassing. What happened to our son was in the local newspaper and on the local news. It felt like the end of the world. We heard about people in public places talking about how terrible our son was. Some of his friends' mothers would no longer allow their sons to associate with him. This was devastating for our son. The incident had involved the destruction of public property, but he had not hurt anyone.

"Our son's psychologist provided a letter for the court, documenting our son's issues and stating his extreme remorse. The judge commended our son for turning himself in. Of course, the local paper did not report *that*.

"Our son's legal troubles cost us a lot financially. We had to settle with an insurance company on our son's behalf, as well as pay court costs. People told us, 'Let him deal with it and pay the price. Let him go to jail. It will teach him a lesson.' But what are you going to do? He was dealing with mental health issues. He drank to hide the pain and did something very impulsive. We are his parents. We know him better than anyone, and we also have to live with the consequences. There is no right answer for this. We had to go by 'What can we live with?' We felt he was remorseful, he needed help, and so we helped him."

A crisis can also represent an opportunity—a turning point—for a family, as Jackie discovered when a judge ordered an assessment for her son David, who had been refusing treatment.

"The only way we even got David into this [treatment] facility was because of a very compassionate judge. Instead of just letting David out on probation again, he decided to ask the prosecutor to get in touch with me so he could talk to me before making a decision. One Friday afternoon at 4:00 P.M., I once again told our story, but this time to a judge who, to this day, I believe was an angel. The judge very kindly and compassionately spoke to my son and said he would like him to see a doctor for 30 days to get assessed, and if, after 30 days, the doctor felt everything was okay—like my son kept saying over and over again he was—he would be released. At 5:00 P.M. on a Friday afternoon, that judge made the prosecutor and the defense attorney make phone calls to get David into the proper safe facility, as opposed to jail, where he was very worried he would be hurt. It was unbelievable and, to this day, I believe that man saved my son's life."

Mary recalls a crisis that arose when her daughter Fiona made a 911 call to police.

"The police responded when Fiona was 13 and reacting very poorly to a medication for joint pain she had been prescribed on top of her psychiatric meds. She threatened her father and siblings with a knife and then called 911 herself. She was taken to the hospital by ambulance at the insistence of police, even though she had calmed down and the situation was under control by the time they arrived. The police officer had no understanding of mental illness. He appeared young and inexperienced. The incident was hard on Fiona and the family. It reinforced for her that she is different and unstable, and it contributed to my wariness about involving police in matters involving individuals with mental illness."

Concerned about such a scenario playing out between police and his son, Dawson, Mark decided to make contact with his local police department ahead of time: "We contacted the police station almost 2 years ago and spoke to someone from the young offenders' division," he recalls. "In our area, they have a team that specializes in children with developmental disabilities and mental health. We gave them our information, including some general information about Dawson so that the team would have the information they needed to respond appropriately, should they ever need to."

That's the essence of crisis planning: anticipating your child's needs in the event of a crisis and doing the necessary planning now, while you have the dual advantages of time and a clear head.

As you begin to think through possible scenarios and identify your child's needs, you'll want to start drafting a crisis plan that includes:

- Emergency contacts (police, ambulance, crisis psychiatric resources)
- Contact information for other people you could call on for help and what you could ask them to do
- A medical emergency information sheet for your child that includes:
  - Your child's full legal name (and the name she prefers to use in conversation, if there's a difference)
  - Your child's health card/insurance policy number and claims contact information
  - Allergy information

o  Medication information (both current medications and medications that have been tried in the past, including details about side
   effects and effectiveness)
o  What techniques are most effective in calming your child when
   she is agitated or upset
o  Contact information for your family physician, your child's therapist, and other key members of your child's mental health care
   team
o  Details about any extended health care benefits coverage you may
   have

Be sure to discuss the contents of your emergency plan with everyone
who is involved in the plan, including your child. And make a point of
reviewing and updating your crisis plan on a regular basis.

## Communicating with Your Child during a Crisis

If your child becomes extremely agitated or upset, or her communication
abilities are in some way impaired during a crisis, you may have to adjust
your communication patterns to ensure that she can calm down enough to
be able to understand what you are trying to say to her.

Woolis suggests the following modifications in *When Someone You Love
Has a Mental Illness*:

- If your child is distracted and experiencing difficulty concentrating,
  keep your messages simple and to the point.
- If your child is anxious or afraid, respond with calmness and reassurance.
- If your child is experiencing rapid mood swings, remain calm and
  try not to take your child's words or actions personally.
- If your child is depressed and withdrawn, assume responsibility for
  initiating conversations and keeping the conversation going.
- If your child is saying things that don't make any sense, resist the
  temptation to argue or to try to talk your child out of her delusions.
  Instead, try to steer the conversation back into more neutral territory.
- If your child is agitated or upset, focus on remaining calm and in
  control, protecting yourself and others from injury, ensuring that
  your child can retreat to a safe space, acknowledging and validating
  your child's feelings, and expressing your desire to help.

## Hopes and Dreams Revisited

During the early days of your child's struggles, when you were uncertain what you were dealing with and what a particular diagnosis might mean for your child's life, you may have found it necessary to put your hopes and dreams for your child on hold. You were too busy dealing with the chaos of the present, and grieving for what might have been, for you to allow yourself to imagine what could be.

At some point as you begin to embrace the possibility of recovery, you may find yourself reinvesting in hopes and dreams for your child once again. Those hopes and dreams will be every bit as unique as you and your child, and they will reflect what you've learned and how you've been affected by your journey so far.

"At first, I wanted the anxiety problems eliminated forever," says Alison, mother of Charlotte. "Now I know that's unrealistic. Now I just want her to be so clearly and easily able to overcome her anxiety that she almost automatically uses one of the coping methods she's learned. That way, when her anxiety crops up, it does not prevent her from doing anything she wants to do (small or large) and she does not require medication, like I do."

"I just want Tom to be happy and to continue to march to his own drummer, recognizing that it is important to keep a steady beat sometimes," says Kim. Tom has been diagnosed with ADHD as well as a learning disability. "At the ripe old age of 11, Tom has a good developing sense of self and has developed some good coping strategies that can be used at home and at school. I hope that this continues for Tom into his teen and adult years. When Tom was little, I just hoped that he wouldn't have any more temper tantrums and that he would make friends. We are getting there, as his temper has really changed and he has a great group of friends."

"My hope for him is that he will be more at ease with his world, that he will be less reclusive, that he will be happy and healthy, that he will function successfully in society, that he will one day be able to live on his own with support (in a group home)," says Betty of her son Stephen, who has been diagnosed with autism and developmental delays.

"Our hope now is that David will stay connected to good professional care throughout his life," says Andrew. "We hope he recovers further than he has to date. We hope that he stays safe and doesn't encounter ignorant and cruel people who might abuse or harm him. We hope he can enjoy some aspects of friendship. We hope he can find ways to enjoy life in healthy ways. We hope he will always have some sense of being connected to family and friends who will continue to care about him. We hope he can be around us in peaceful ways and enjoy some family life with all of us.

These goals or dreams have evolved over time as we've come to grips with the limitations of his recovery and his ongoing level of functioning. We stay open to and hopeful of further recovery."

"I hope that my sons find a way to move forward without the stigma hanging over them," says Michelle, mother of John and Martin. "I hope they find the supports and strength to figure out the strategies that work to allow them to be productive, contributing, positive members of society. I hope they find peace. I hope they find life partners who understand and support them."

"My hope is that Dawson will find inner happiness, that the demons he has wrestled with from his past—his tragedies and life before us—will no longer have such control over his life," says Mark. "I hope he finds love and is able to love back. I hope that he is happy and independent. I dream of the day when he is able to stand on his own two feet and be proud of what he has accomplished."

For Eve, daring to dream about the future means letting go of the pain and regret of the past—a process that continues, even as her three daughters move into adulthood. "I'm still trying to learn to let go and not take their rejection of my help personally. I remind myself that they have a right to their own life, and they have the right to mess it up, just like I did. I messed up my life in different, less dangerous ways when I was their age, but I learned from my mistakes, and I hope they do, too. One social worker told me that kids with mental illness often pull it together around age 30, if they're going to. She said that's when they decide they need to take their medication or make up with their parents or get their lives together, in general. I try to keep this perspective in mind. I try to remember that the story isn't over yet, and it won't be for a long time. They'll keep living and hopefully growing long after my life is over, most likely. They are going to have to find their own way. As much as I'd like to (and tried to), I can't do that for them."

"Do parents ever stop dreaming for their children?" asks Claire, mother of Owen. "It is our hope that he will recognize his need for treatment and go on to have a fulfilling life. We dream that someday he will go back to school and have a career. We hope that one day he will marry someone who will understand and support him. We think he will make a wonderful dad. We are not there yet, but we hope and pray that [we will be] someday."

## Endings and Beginnings

When your child was first diagnosed, you may have felt like the world was ending.

Now you understand that while your child's diagnosis may have brought one chapter of your life to an end, receiving the insights that accompanied that diagnosis also sparked a new beginning for you and your child.

"I view our lives as a gift," says Meg, whose son, Jayden, has been diagnosed with an anxiety disorder (but who is likely on the autism spectrum). "Jayden and I are on a journey together. There is a reason why all this has happened. He is here to teach me. Our journey will give us the means to educate and advocate for others. This experience has challenged me to be patient and creative."

Priya shares that perspective: "The experience was both a trial by fire and an incredible period of growth," she notes, reflecting on the circumstances surrounding her son's Asperger syndrome diagnosis. "Our son wasn't the only person to emerge from this process a stronger and better person. . . . If you can come to a place of peace, it's amazing what you as a person can gain from this, too."

Part of what you stand to gain is a warmer, more connected relationship with your child—the result of having weathered powerful storms together. "I find that I have a much closer relationship with Sophie than I might otherwise have had," says Sandra, whose daughter Sophie has been diagnosed with moderate autism with global developmental delays. "Because I have had to learn to read her so well, we are very much in tune with one another."

You might also find that your compassion for others increases exponentially. "Skyler's diagnoses have impacted my work as a teacher," says Leigh, whose son has been diagnosed with ADHD, anxiety, and depression. "I began to see youth who struggled with mental health issues in a whole new way. I understood better that what they were experiencing was way beyond their control. I understood that there was no easy solution. I was more willing to work cooperatively with them and their parents to see what we could do together to get through the school piece. I knew that sometimes school was the last thing on a kid's mind. I also began to gain a true understanding of the lack of resources available to parents and educators, including those that would put health on the front burner and school on the back if necessary."

"I learned that I'm stronger than I thought, that I can handle more than I thought, that mental illness doesn't have to be a permanent condition or to hold you back from achieving your goals, that mental illness doesn't define you (although it is part of you like anything else)," says Mara, whose son, Jake, has been diagnosed with ADHD and whose daughter, Samantha, has been diagnosed with anxiety. "I also learned not to rest until I got what I needed for my child and not to be shy or embarrassed to ask questions."

Andrew, father of David, says that the biggest challenge for him has been "balancing the lifelong worry generated by the child's vulnerability with the challenge of preserving one's sense of wonder and joy of living." He has chosen to embrace the lessons that can be learned because of what he has experienced alongside his son. "If we stay open to the opportunities and invitations to learn and grow, we have the unique option of experiencing some good things we would never have experienced had we not been faced with the challenges brought to us by our child."

As Vincent van Gogh wrote so long ago, "There is peace even in the storm."

# 14

# Creating a Better System

It's hard to see the forest for the trees when you are caught up with helping and advocating for your child. But the experience might leave you feeling that the system currently in place to help you and your family is not delivering everything it might. *I must be doing something wrong,* you may be thinking. *Surely it can't be this difficult to make the system work for my child.*

Based on my own experiences trying to get the health care system and the school system to work for my own four children, my gut instinct is telling me this: it's not you; it's the system, or rather systems, that have the problem.

> Navigating health care is similar to trying to navigate the legal system or political system. It has a language and culture unique to itself.
> —**Cat, mother of two teenagers with mental health challenges**

It's important for you to understand this so that you don't start blaming yourself for not being efficient enough or persistent enough or smart enough or *whatever-else* enough to fix the mental health care system and educational systems on your own.

Perhaps you'll feel a little better if I share an example or two of some of the crazy—and crazy-making—things we have dealt with as a family over the years. Here are two of the highlights (or lowlights) that remain at the top of my mind.

We were invited to a meeting at our children's elementary school so that the principal could propose a "modified schedule" for our son Erik, who had been diagnosed with ADHD and ODD and who was in grade 3 at the time. The principal proposed that Erik be "allowed" to attend school for half an hour a day, from 9:00 to 9:30 A.M. We respectfully declined the offer.

We tried to make sense of a local youth mental health agency's decision to have young people initially connect with an outreach worker and then switch to a permanent counselor. Our daughter, who was in her early teens at the time, became quite attached to the outreach worker (hey, attachment *happens*), and she did not want to switch to the permanent counselor. The agency was not willing or able to accommodate her request. Julie went through the motions of going to her counseling appointments with the new counselor, but she took every opportunity to express her extreme displeasure with the entire process. I still have a picture in my head of dropping her off at one of her appointments while she was sporting an Emily the Strange T-shirt that read, "My problem is YOU."

In the interest of fairness, I should add that we also managed to connect with some amazing mental health care professionals, principals, vice principals, teachers, and coaches who made a point of connecting with and caring about my kids. They each made a huge difference in the lives of my children and our family. They also showed me what truly great care looks and feels like. Frankly, no child should have to settle for anything less.

When things are not so great (when you've just run up against the most nonsensical, non-family-friendly policy imaginable), it is all too easy to get caught up in feeling angry about the many ways the system keeps getting it wrong. But that won't change anything. Sure, it's important to express those feelings—which is why we all need friends who will listen, hug us, and give us the courage to keep on keeping on. But at some point we have to switch back into action mode. That means focusing on making positive change for our own children and other children, and allowing ourselves to imagine a future that isn't just better but that is actually quite awesome.

So, what do we want? What would make for a better mental health care system for children and youth and their families?

## A System That Emphasizes Prevention and Early Treatment

Our greatest opportunity to help children and families is in the area of prevention and early treatment. According to Active Minds, half of all serious adult psychiatric illnesses emerge by age 14 and three-quarters are present by age 25. It makes so much more sense to either prevent problems from occurring or to treat these problems right away than it does to attempt to deal with the financial and societal fallout after the fact. After all, children whose mental health difficulties go untreated are likely to go on to become teenagers and then adults with mental health problems. Providing support to parents who are struggling (who are dealing with parental depression or living in poverty, for example) and improving access to early childhood mental health assessments (to identify children who would benefit from early treatment) are just two ways that children's outcomes could be improved, and the lifetime costs associated with mental illness and disability could be reduced.

And, of course, the same principle applies to children who are struggling with neurodevelopmental disorders, like autism spectrum disorder, and behavioral disorders, like ODD: early interventions that build upon the child and the family's strengths can change the entire life trajectory for that child. As Liza Long, mental health advocate and author of *The Price of Silence,* puts it: "We know that if we can get kids the right interventions early, they can have great lives."

This kind of emphasis on early intervention makes sense to Kristina, whose daughter, Clare, has been diagnosed with bipolar disorder and general anxiety disorder as well as food sensitivities and irritable bowel syndrome. It's a matter of preventing a small problem from snowballing into something much bigger, she explains: "So many seemingly bad behaviors are actually maladaptive coping mechanisms and [if left untreated] they can spiral from there."

Early childhood screening for mental health should be something that happens automatically during well-child checkups with pediatricians and other primary care providers, in the same way that children are automatically screened for problems related to physical development. Clearly there's plenty of room for improvement on this front. A 2008 poll conducted by the C. S. Mott Children's Hospital found that 56% of parents report that their child's primary care doctor never asked whether they had any concerns about their child's mental health. Not once.

> I'd also like to see it possible for more intensive treatment to be made available (and paid for by insurance companies) early on. We wasted years (and many thousands of dollars of our—and our health providers'—money) pursuing treatments that were too infrequent and not intensive enough. I believe that if our three children with mental health issues had been able to get intensive trauma treatment (residential, partial-residential, day treatment, or outpatient) early on, we would have saved tens of thousands of dollars, and their great suffering (and ours) could have been significantly minimized.
>
> **—Eve, mother of three daughters who have all dealt with adoption-related trauma and behavioral issues**

So what can we do to make early childhood screening for mental illness the new normal?

We can ensure that everyone who works with children—health care providers and educators alike—receives proper training about the early warning signs of mental illness so that potential mental health problems can be flagged right away. Ideally, these types of conversations should be nonalarmist, supportive, and completely matter of fact, adopting the same kind of tone a teacher would use when flagging a potential vision problem for a parent. "We need to be able to say to parents, 'We've done these standard assessments at school, and we're concerned about your child. Here's why we're concerned, and here are the resources that are available to you,'" notes mental health advocate Andrew Solomon, author of *Far from the Tree: Parents, Children, and the Search for Identity*.

## A System That Makes Sense to Families

Figuring out how to navigate the children's mental health system is no easy task, as any parent who has been there, tried to do that, can tell you.

The 2008 parent survey mentioned above found, for example, that 46% of parents of children with a mental health diagnosis had difficulty accessing mental health services for their child, either because it was difficult to find a provider (46%), treatment was unaffordable (43%), there were long waiting lists for an appointment (35%), or they didn't know where to turn for help (35%).

Rebecca has experienced this frustration firsthand in her effort to obtain the right combination of services for her daughter, Madalyn, who has been diagnosed with a learning disability and is currently undergoing a series of other assessments. "It seems ridiculous to go one place to get a psychoeducational assessment, then to another place to get services for a kid with anxiety/learning disabilities, and then somewhere else for an assessment for occupational therapy."

Jennifer, whose daughter deals with physical and psychological difficulties related to tuberous sclerosis, echoes that call for more integrated care: "The absolutely complete disconnect between medical professionals who treat physical problems and those who treat mental/emotional problems is such a challenge. All of Jessica's problems are interlinked. You cannot separate one from the other, but the health care system in this country is so fragmented that she has probably ten different specialists handling different parts of her, which is beyond ridiculous."

At the heart of the problem is the fact that the system isn't really a system—at least, not in any meaningful sense of the word. Children's services are scattered across a variety of different sectors (public health, education, child protection, and justice, for example) and jurisdictions (including federal, state, and county). And, of course, there is a dizzying mix of public and private—insured and uninsured—treatments on offer as well. Is it any wonder that simply figuring out what types of services are available continues to be a major challenge—and that wraparound care (having a single care plan in place for each child who needs one, as opposed to multiple care plans from different health care providers) continues to be so elusive?

And then there's the fact that the system sometimes seems to be better equipped to meet the needs of those providing the care than of those actually accessing the care—namely families and children. Services need to be offered at times that work for children and families (after school, during evenings, and on weekends) and in locations that are comfortable and convenient for them (at home or in school-based mental health treatment hubs, for example).

When doctors and other experts don't know what's behind a child's behavior, parents can find themselves being forced to reject "innuendo or frank assertions that it might be their parenting or their own emotional problem that is creating the challenges for their child," says Stan Kutcher, a professor in the Department of Psychiatry at Dalhousie University in Nova Scotia, Canada.

What parents want is not to be blamed but rather to be treated as partners in their children's care—and to be provided with the support and information they need to provide suitable care for their child.

Things tend to get complicated once children reach the point at which they become capable of making their own medical decisions. It's a case of patients' rights and privacy concerns colliding with parents' hardwired desires to care for their children. "Your child can refuse treatment, and health care professionals will not give you any information unless your child allows it," explains Claire, whose son Owen has been diagnosed with bipolar disorder, a personality disorder, and extreme anxiety. "This is really frustrating. You're left caring for your son or daughter but may not be allowed to be part of the treatment process."

Parents like Claire need good information to continue to provide good care to their children who are struggling with mental illness, and yet they find themselves stuck between a legal rock and a parental hard place.

"Our son is on-again and off-again regarding prescribed treatments [counseling and medication]. This continues to be the most frustrating, bewildering experience as a parent. We worry all the time. We can always tell when he is off his medication. We get endless phone calls. He gets quite manic and impulsive in his behavior. The law does not side with the family, only the individual rights of the patient, even when you have your son's best interest in mind."

Liza Long understands those feelings of frustration—and agrees that the law needs to do a better job of taking into account both the needs of the family *and* the needs of the child. "This has become a social justice issue for me."

## A System That Provides Suitable Supports
## to Young Adults

The young adult years are a time of transition. The challenge, as many families quickly discover, is finding and tapping into suitable supports as young people "age out of" services and supports that were available to them when they were younger—and finding a way to pay for the supports that the young person needs in order to thrive.

Part of the problem is that there simply aren't as many supports available.

Linda, whose son, Sam, has been diagnosed with ADHD and learning disabilities, explains: "Our son was unable to obtain a high school diploma or to attend college. He participated in vocational programs and got a certificate indicating that he'd completed high school. It was difficult to figure out what to do with him after that. There is a shortage of programs for young adults with mental illness."

Jennifer confirms that observation: "Right now I'm working on what Jess will be doing after high school, and everyone assumes that there are programs for that. Well, tell me where to sign up for them because I don't see them anywhere. One local program, for job coaching, has a 6-year waiting list. It might as well not exist at all, as far as helping Jess is concerned."

And then there's the issue of cost. The need to keep reaching for your own wallet to meet your child's needs well into adulthood can be a source of considerable stress for parents. You may be forced to tap into your own retirement savings and/or remortgage your home in order to meet your adult child's needs today. That might mean subsidizing the cost of his apartment, providing him with grocery money during times of unemployment (or underemployment), and/or covering other hefty out-of-pocket expenses, including medication, therapy, and ambulance rides. While some young adults are able to qualify for disability payments through Social Security or for medical assistance through Medicaid, "Families in crisis due to mental health issues get very limited help given the costs associated with mental health care," notes Bob, whose son Steve has been diagnosed with bipolar disorder.

And, of course, there can be other unanticipated expenses.

Carolyn is still reeling from the financial hit her family took when her son Ezra ran into trouble with the law: "While I'm glad we hired the lawyer, paying that fee is something that set off a ripple we haven't and may never recover from—but that's the lengths you go to when your kid needs you. It would have been great to know where to turn or to have had help that wasn't so expensive."

## A System That Works for People
## Who Are Struggling with Dual Diagnosis

Children and adolescents who are dealing with substance abuse problems as well as mental health challenges need access to nonjudgmental treatment and care that recognizes that when mental health and addiction problems occur together, they must be treated together; that treats addiction as a chronic health issue as opposed to a moral or criminal issue; and that doesn't insist that a child or adolescent be "clean" (drug-free) to access treatment. We now know that common genetic factors may leave individuals vulnerable to both mental disorders and addiction disorders—or to experiencing a second disorder once the first has appeared—and that environmental factors like stress and trauma may act as triggers. When addiction and mental health challenges occur, families must be included in assessment and treatment; and postrecovery treatment care options must be put in place to ensure continued recovery.

## A System That Is Adequately Funded—
## and That Funds the Right Treatments

According to the Bazelon Center for Mental Health Law, "Mental disorders affect about one in five American children, yet only about a fifth of these children actually receive the mental health services they need." At the heart of the problem is a critical shortage of child psychiatrists and other mental health professionals—and the fact that children's mental health services tend to be chronically underfunded: "While many communities have begun to build systems of care, they often receive too little funding and serve far fewer children than is necessary," it notes.

And then there's the fact that we keep investing our precious mental health care dollars in the wrong types of treatments—crisis supports as opposed to the community-based supports that allow children and families to thrive. "Despite a virtual consensus among experts that residential treatment is an archaic and ineffective approach, nearly a quarter of national spending on children's mental health goes to this form of institutional care," notes the Bazelon Center. "It is time to stop this misguided investment and instead invest in building a foundation of supportive services that allows children with mental disorders to thrive in their communities."

Darcy Gruttadaro, director of the NAMI Child and Adolescent Action Center, agrees that a shift in funding priorities is needed. "We are a very crisis-driven system. We wait for a crisis to hit, and then families have very few options: you can go to the ER; you can call the police. We don't have mobile crisis intervention units in a lot of communities. We don't have school-based crisis care. . . . So, in many cases, kids are being diverted into the juvenile justice system, whether they've committed an offense or not."

> I want less stigma so my child can have friends, people who will watch out for him, not hurt him. I want support so that my other children don't have to suffer. I want my husband to understand why I have to help our son, because no one else will. I want more providers, better access, better payments. I want the school to be more helpful and earlier. . . . I don't want you to suspend my first grader for terroristic threatening because he threw a piece of paper and said "I hate you" to the teacher. . . . I want the criminal justice system and police to know how to cope with mental illness. I want people to know you can look "normal" and still need help.
> 
> —Carolyn, whose son Ezra has been diagnosed with pervasive developmental delay, ADHD, anxiety, and depression and whose daughter Norah has been diagnosed with sensory processing disorder

We need to stop criminalizing people, including children, with mental illness out of some misguided notion that this is the best or the only way to keep them safe, she stresses. Instead, we need to prevent kids from entering the so-called "school-to-prison pipeline" by providing more and better community-based supports. That includes crisis intervention teams made up of police officers who have received special training on how to deescalate situations involving people experiencing a mental health crisis.

It also means funding evidence-based treatments: treatments with a proven track record for making a difference. After all, it's not good enough to merely offer a child access to treatment. You need to offer that child access to the right treatment. Gruttadaro explains: "What I want to say to policymakers is 'Enough on just access. What are people getting? What is the quality of care? How do we know it's good? Are we tracking outcomes?

Are we looking at our data? Are we making sure that what we're delivering is a research-based intervention (whenever we know that research exists to address that condition)?'"

"We need to make this a public health priority because we're paying for these kids in all the wrong places," adds Gruttadaro. "We are paying far more than we need to and we're interrupting their ability to ultimately be independent, productive adults in society—and there's a tremendous cost to that. And the impact on families and communities—their productivity and the devastation they experience—is also tremendous."

Liza Long would also welcome that kind of dialogue. "This is a public health crisis, and we're treating it like it's just bad choices and bad parenting. That's not what it is at all. It's a public health crisis, so why aren't we treating it that way and throwing all kinds of resources at the problem when we know what works? We would save an enormous amount of money, but it's so much bigger than that. We would also save so many lives."

> Sam has been in at least five residential programs, none of which were very effective. I wish we had known to ask questions about the training and credentials of staff, as we later learned that most of the onsite staff, especially at night and on weekends, were untrained and undereducated.
> —Linda, mother of Sam, who has been diagnosed with ADHD and learning disabilities

In the end, it all comes down to what type of society we want to be.

If you agree that we can do better—that we must do better—when it comes to child and youth mental health, there's plenty you can do to work for change.

## Write Letters

You can write to politicians in your community, speaking out for the need for more and better child and youth mental health care, and send copies of your letters to your local newspaper to spark a dialogue.

## Work in Partnership

You can join forces with advocacy groups like NAMI (*www.nami.org*) and the National Federation of Families for Children's Mental Health (*www.ffcmh.org*) that are working to make things better for children and families. See the website for this book (*www.anndouglas.net*) to find out about the important work being done by other advocacy groups too.

## Speak Out

Talk to friends and coworkers about your family's experiences and ask them to raise their voices too. There is strength in numbers.

## Moving Forward

Staying focused on feeling empowered and making positive strides will keep the feelings of helplessness at bay. Remember that you can make a difference—for your child, for your family, and for your community.

# Epilogue
## After the Storm

If this were a fairy tale, this would be the part where we'd get to the "happily ever after." But life isn't a fairy tale, is it? And even though my life will never be fairy-tale perfect (how boring would that be?), I have to admit it's pretty amazing.

Consider this email I received from my son Scott's first employer shortly after he landed his first job in (you guessed it) the computer industry: "I have the honor and pleasure of working with [Scott] every day. . . . He is so well grounded. . . . He has an incredible curiosity that is a joy to feed and witness. You have done a remarkable job raising that fine young man."

This kind of awesomeness isn't confined to just one of my children, I should add.

Erik scooped up an award from his professional association at his recent university graduation. And he's holding down two (count 'em, two!) jobs in his chosen profession. Julie has started submitting her photography to a number of juried art competitions this year—an act of courage that would have been unthinkable for her not that long ago. And, in the interest of full disclosure, allow me to tell you this part: she's been rocking the competitions. And my son Ian recently launched his own small-engine repair business, at age 16. He's demonstrated remarkable self-awareness and business acumen. In fact, many budding entrepreneurs might want to adopt his technique of prescreening potential clients and heading off those who are likely to be a pain in the butt: "I'm sorry. I don't think this is going to work out. Good luck finding someone else to work on your snowblower."

As you can see, all of my children are thriving in their own way. I couldn't be prouder. But what leaves me feeling incredibly happy at the end of the day is the fact that we continue to be a close, connected, and loving family. We managed to weather the stormiest of times—times that could have torn our family apart.

That's not to say that the storm clouds have receded permanently. I still keep a watchful eye on the horizon. I suppose I always will. But even if the dark clouds return (as they well may) and one of us ends up struggling with mental illness once again, I know we will continue to find our way together.

> There is no health without mental health.
>
> —World Health Organization

We've come so far.

We've learned so much.

We have been strengthened by the storm.

# Appendix A

# Glossary

*504 plan:* A plan that spells out the accommodations that must be made for a student whose disability "substantially" limits his ability to participate in school. Such a plan is mandated by Section 504 of the Rehabilitation Act, a federal law that protects the rights of individuals with disabilities in programs and activities that receive funding from the U.S. Department of Education.

*acceptance and commitment therapy (ACT):* A type of therapy that encourages individuals to live their lives mindfully and in accordance with their values. It emphasizes acceptance, mindfulness, and behavioral change.

*addiction:* The term used to describe physical or psychological dependence. *See also* substance abuse.

*adjustment disorder:* A disorder that occurs when a child has extreme difficulty coping with (or adjusting to) a change in circumstance (a major life change, loss, or stressful event).

*Americans with Disabilities Act (ADA):* The ADA is a federal law that prohibits discrimination against individuals with disabilities in a wide range of settings, including both public and private schools.

*amygdala:* An almond-shaped set of neurons in the brain, responsible for processing emotional memories, managing responses to fear, and readying the body for action.

*anhedonia:* The absence of enjoyment or pleasure. A common symptom of depression.

*anorexia nervosa:* A type of eating disorder. It is characterized by an extreme fear of gaining weight, persistent efforts to restrict calorie intake, and distorted beliefs about body weight or shape. Approximately 0.4% of young women

237

struggle with anorexia nervosa. The disorder is 10 times as common in women as in men.

*anxiety:* An emotion that is characterized by worry and tension and that may include physical symptoms such as a dry mouth, a rapid heartbeat, sweating, dizziness, nausea, and diarrhea.

*anxiety disorder:* A group of mental disorders that are characterized by excessive fear and anxiety and related behavioral disturbances. Many anxiety disorders develop in childhood and, if not treated, persist into adulthood. They are twice as likely to occur in females as in males. See Appendix C for details about some specific anxiety disorders.

*applied behavior analysis (ABA):* A therapy for children with autism that combines close observation of the child's existing behaviors with positive prompts or reinforcements in an effort to increase desired behaviors.

*art therapy:* A therapeutic process that incorporates art activities into the treatment process. Art therapy has been proven to be helpful in treating posttraumatic stress disorder (PTSD), behavioral disorders, mood disorders, and problems with self-esteem.

*Asperger syndrome:* An autism spectrum disorder named after Hans Asperger, a Vienna-based pediatrician who identified the cluster of symptoms that is now associated with his name. People with Asperger syndrome typically face social and communication challenges, exhibit inappropriate behavior, and may face other related challenges (anxiety, depression, attentional difficulties, tics or Tourette syndrome, gross- and fine-motor skills deficits, poor organizational skills). People with Asperger syndrome are generally of above-average intelligence. *Note:* Asperger syndrome is no longer classified as a separate type of autism, as of the fifth edition of the *Diagnostic and Statistical Manual of Mental Disorders* (DSM-5). This decision was quite controversial.

*assessment:* An information-gathering process that allows a mental health professional to come to a decision about a diagnosis. The assessment process may include interviews with you and your child; detailed questionnaires dealing with your child's medical history, developmental history, and behavior (to be completed by you, your child's other parent, and your child's teacher); a history of any physical or psychological traumas (natural disaster, a death in the family); a family history of mental, neurodevelopmental, or behavioral disorders; a review of reports from your child's school; and psychological testing for your child.

*attachment:* The connection between parent and child that allows the child to feel safe, secure, protected, and comforted. As humans, we are wired for emotional connection with others. When our relationship connections are supportive, we feel comforted, and our brains become trained in such a way that we become capable of comforting ourselves.

*attachment-based family therapy (ABFT):* A type of therapy designed to resolve attachment problems in children. It is based on the beliefs that attachment problems can be resolved, parents can learn to be more responsive to their children's needs, and children with attachment problems can learn how to trust and communicate with their parents. ABFT has been proven to reduce the severity of depression and anxiety symptoms, feelings of hopelessness, and suicidal thoughts, and to encourage healthy parent–child relationships.

*attention-deficit/hyperactivity disorder (ADHD):* A neurodevelopmental disorder that affects a child's ability to regulate his attention, emotions, and behavior. There are three separate subtypes of ADHD: the primarily hyperactive–impulsive subtype (which is quite rare), the primarily inattentive subtype (formerly known as attention-deficit disorder), and the combined subtype (the most common type of ADHD, made up of individuals who exhibit symptoms of hyperactivity, impulsivity, and inattention). See Appendix C for further details.

*autism spectrum disorder (ASD):* An umbrella term used to describe a range of complex neurodevelopmental disorders that are characterized by social impairments, communication difficulties, and repetitive patterns of behavior. The incidence of autism was 1 in 68 children in 2010, according to the CDC; DSM-5 reports an incidence rate of approximately 1%. Males are four times as likely to be diagnosed with an autism spectrum disorder as females.

*behavioral activation (BA):* A treatment for depression that encourages people to participate in activities, even if they don't feel like it, so that they can break free of the cycle of avoidance and withdrawal that can quickly start feeding upon itself when someone is depressed. The aim of the therapy is to help the person make the connection between being involved in activities that they enjoy and improved mood.

*bipolar disorder:* A type of mood disorder. See Appendix C for details.

*borderline personality disorder:* A type of personality disorder. *See also* personality disorder.

*brief- or solution-focused therapy:* A type of therapy that focuses on the identification and achievement of personal goals.

*bulimia nervosa:* A type of eating disorder. It is characterized by recurrent episodes of binge eating; attempts to prevent weight gain by engaging in unhealthy behaviors such as self-induced vomiting, the misuse of laxatives, diuretics, or other medications, fasting, or excessive exercise; and distorted beliefs about body shape and weight. The incidence of bulimia nervosa is approximately 1 to 1.5% in young women. It is 10 times as common in women as in men.

*circadian rhythm:* The body's internal clock. It operates on a cycle that is (approximately) 24 hours in length and helps to control our sleep–wake patterns, our temperature, and our hormones. A shift in teenagers' circadian rhythms causes them to feel naturally alert late at night, making it difficult for them to get the sleep they need before they have to wake up and go to school. (Teenagers need at least 8½ hours of sleep per day.)

*cognitive-behavioral therapy (CBT):* A type of therapy based on the idea that our thoughts, feelings, and behaviors are all interconnected and that changing our thinking can result in changes to our feelings and our behavior (just as changing our behavior can change the way we think and feel). At a biological level, CBT helps to tame the amygdala (which can get caught up in endless loops of what-if thinking) by focusing on more rational thinking processes (which activate the parts of the brain involved in logic and reason).

*comorbid disorder:* A disorder that exists alongside but is not related to another disorder (as in two types of anxiety).

*compulsions:* Repetitive behaviors or rituals that an individual relies on in an effort to control obsessive thoughts (obsessions).

*conduct disorder (CD):* A type of disruptive, impulse control, and conduct disorder. See Appendix C for details.

*crisis plan:* A detailed plan for handling any potential emergency situation involving your child. It should include emergency contacts, the names of other people you could call on for help in the event of an emergency, and emergency medical information for your child. If your child has reached the age where she is responsible for her own medical decisions, you might also want to talk to her about signing waivers that would allow you to make contact with her doctor and decide upon treatment options if she were too ill to make such decisions herself.

*delusion:* A false belief that someone persists in believing despite evidence to the contrary.

*depression:* A type of mood disorder. See Appendix C for details.

*depressive episode:* A period of depression in major depressive disorder or bipolar disorder.

*desensitization: See* exposure and response prevention therapy (ERP).

*developmental delay:* Sometimes referred to as *intellectual disability.*

*dialectical behavior therapy (DBT):* A type of therapy that builds on the principles of cognitive-behavioral therapy but also focuses on teaching mindfulness (living in the present moment with awareness and acceptance), emotional regulation, distress tolerance, and interpersonal skills through both individual and group therapy. DBT gets its name from the word *dialectical,* which refers to balancing two seemingly contradictory ideas. In this case, DBT involves learning how to hold two seemingly contradictory ideas in your mind at the same time: for example, accepting yourself as you are right now while also committing to work to change yourself. DBT was originally designed as a treatment for borderline personality disorder in women with a history of suicidal tendencies. It has since been adapted to treat other conditions, including eating disorders, depression, substance abuse, and suicidal and self-injurious behaviors.

*disability:* Difficulties or limitations in performing the basic activities of daily living that result from health conditions, including mental disorders. The World Health Organization defines *disability* as follows: "Disabilities is an umbrella term, covering impairments, activity limitations, and participation restrictions. An impairment is a problem in body function or structure; an activity limitation is a difficulty encountered by an individual in executing a task or action; while a participation restriction is a problem experienced by an individual in involvement in life situations."

*disruptive, impulse control, and conduct disorders:* Disorders that involve problems with the regulation (or self-control) of emotions and behavior. See Appendix C for details about two such disorders: conduct disorder and oppositional defiant disorder.

*dopamine:* A neurotransmitter (or "brain messenger") that is involved in learning, reward, attention, and movement.

*dual diagnosis:* The term used when someone is diagnosed with a mental illness and a substance use disorder.

*Early Start Denver Model:* A play-based early intervention specifically developed for very young children with autism. It is equally applicable to home and day care settings, and can be offered in groups or one-on-one.

*effective behavior support (EBS):* Sometimes called *positive behavior support (PBS).* EBS is designed to reduce undesirable behaviors and is typically offered in a school setting. A functional assessment is conducted to determine why a particular behavior is occurring and to come up with a plan for responding to the problem behavior while teaching the child new skills that will allow the child to behave more effectively or appropriately.

*epigenetics:* The study of how genes are expressed through interaction with the environment.

*exposure and response prevention therapy (ERP):* A type of behavioral therapy that involves exposing the child in a controlled setting and in a controlled manner to things that trigger his anxiety so that he can gradually learn to tolerate those feelings. This type of therapy can help children who struggle with obsessive–compulsive disorder, social anxiety, specific phobias, panic disorder, and generalized anxiety disorder. Also known as *exposure therapy, desensitization,* and *systematic desensitization.*

*eye movement desensitization and reprocessing (EMDR):* A type of therapy that involves stimulating the brain through eye movements and that is designed to reduce the intensity of distressing memories associated with past traumas.

*family therapy:* A generic term used to describe any sort of therapy that you participate in as a family (as opposed to therapy that involves your child only, or that limits you to the role of support person). Most treatment plans for children and adolescents recommend family therapy, because it gives family members an opportunity to discuss and work on issues that are affecting the entire family, like how to deal with a family member's mental illness.

*FAPE:* Free appropriate public education. The Rehabilitation Act and the Individuals with Disabilities Education Act uphold the right of students with disabilities to a "free appropriate public education."

*FERPA:* The Family Educational Rights and Privacy Act—federal privacy legislation governing student educational records.

*FMLA:* The Family and Medical Leave Act, which allows eligible employees of employers who are covered by the act to take unpaid, job-protected leave for up to 12 weeks in each 12-month period to care for a family member with "a serious health condition"—and which mandates that group health insurance coverage be continued for such employees "under the same terms and conditions as if the employee had not taken leave."

*frontal lobe:* The part of the brain that is responsible for controlling movement and planning our behavior, and for other complex tasks like reasoning and problem solving. It is also home to our personality and our emotions.

*group therapy:* Therapy that happens in a group setting. Members of the group are typically working to resolve the same or related issues.

*hallucination:* When the brain senses something as being real though it isn't, in fact, real (for example, hearing voices when no one has spoken).

*hippocampus:* The part of the brain that translates emotional information into memory. It is also involved in regulating our emotions.

*hypnotherapy:* A type of therapy that involves inducing a state of deep relaxation and an altered state of consciousness. People with anxiety disorders tend to respond well to hypnotherapy.

*hypomania:* A milder form of mania. Unlike a full-blown mania, hypomania does not include full-fledged hallucinations.

*individualized education plan (IEP):* A document that outlines program adaptations or modifications and other supports that will be made by your child's school because of your child's special needs. An IEP should be jointly developed by the parents and the school and reviewed and updated at least once per year.

*Individuals with Disabilities Education Act (IDEA):* IDEA is a federal law that guarantees each child the right to a free appropriate public education that meets her needs for education and related services in the "least restrictive environment" possible.

*inpatient services:* Services that are provided to an individual who is staying in hospital.

*interpersonal psychotherapy (IPT):* Therapy that focuses on relationships with family and friends. With this type of therapy, a child is encouraged to consider how relationships with other people can affect his moods and behavior—and how his moods and behavior can, in turn, affect his relationships with other people. IPT is frequently used to treat depression in children and adolescents.

*manic phase:* One of the two phases experienced by people with bipolar disorder (the other being the depressive phase).

*mental disorder:* A disturbance in thinking, emotions, and perception that is severe enough to affect day-to-day functioning. A mental disorder is a medical illness diagnosed using internationally recognized criteria such as the *Diagnostic and Statistical Manual of Mental Disorders* (DSM) or the *International Classification of Diseases* (ICD). *Mental disorder* means the same thing as *mental illness*.

*mental health:* A state of well-being as opposed to merely the absence of illness. As the World Health Organization notes: "Mental health is defined as a state of well-being in which every individual realizes his or her own potential, can cope with the normal stresses of life, can work productively and fruitfully, and is able to make a contribution to her or his community. . . . Health is a state of complete physical, mental and social well-being and not merely the absence of disease or infirmity."

*mental illness: See* mental disorder.

*mindfulness:* "Paying attention in a particular way: on purpose, in the present moment, and nonjudgmentally," according to Jon Kabat-Zinn, who pioneered the use of mindfulness in therapy and is the founder of the Stress Reduction Clinic at the University of Massachusetts Medical School.

*mindfulness-based therapies:* Treatment approaches that combine therapy with some type of mindfulness meditation. Mindfulness-based cognitive therapy (MBCT) was designed to help people who have experienced recurrent episodes of depression, but it has been applied to other disorders as well. Mindfulness-based stress reduction (MBSR) combines mindfulness meditation with yoga.

*mindful parenting:* A style of parenting that involves active listening, nonjudgmental acceptance of yourself and your child, being aware of your emotions and your child's emotions (and being able to control your emotions in the moment), and having compassion for yourself and your child.

*mood disorders:* A group of mental disorders that relate to the brain's ability to regulate mood. "Everyone experiences 'highs' and 'lows' in life, but people with mood disorders experience them with greater intensity and for longer periods of time than most people," notes the Canadian Mental Health Association. The incidence of mood disorders is 1 in 10. See Appendix C for more information about some specific types of mood disorders.

*motivational interviewing (MI):* A therapeutic technique that helps people address ambivalence about changing their behavior. By eliciting reasons for and against change, therapists help clients get more invested in making changes that make sense to them.

*multisystemic therapy (MST):* An intensive, short-term therapy based on the premise that problem behavior is the result of many interacting factors in many different areas (or systems) of a child's life. It is designed to improve family functioning, promote academic and social skills, encourage healthy peer relationships, and address any other problems that are preventing a child from thriving. MST therapists (who have a small caseload and work with children with severe behavioral problems) are available to families 7 days a week, 24 hours a day.

*music therapy:* The use of music as a therapeutic technique to maximize health and well-being. Music therapy has been demonstrated to be of benefit to children with autism and adolescents with at-risk behaviors, and for treating depression, schizophrenia, and addictions.

*narrative therapy:* A collaborative approach to therapy that involves making sense out of your life through the telling—and reframing—of your own life story.

*neurofeedback:* Sometimes called *electroencephalography (EEG) biofeedback.* A form of computer-guided biofeedback that allows you to regulate your own brainwaves so that they fall within a particular range believed to maximize well-being. Although it lacks strong scientific evidence, neurofeedback has been used to treat a variety of disorders, including ADHD, depression, substance abuse, and PTSD.

*neuropsychology:* The study of the link between the brain and behavior.

*neurotransmitters:* The chemicals that carry messages in the brain. Some of the neurotransmitters that impact thinking, mood, and behavior are serotonin (mood, impulsivity, anger, and aggressiveness), norepinephrine (attention, perception, motivation, and arousal), and dopamine (learning, reward, attention, and movement).

*norepinephrine:* A neurotransmitter (or "brain messenger") that is involved in attention, perception, motivation, and arousal.

*obsessions:* Persistent, unwanted thoughts that cause significant disruption to a person's life.

*oppositional defiant disorder (ODD):* A type of disruptive, impulse control, and conduct disorder. See Appendix C for details.

*panic attack:* Periods of intense fear or anxiety that come on suddenly and can last anywhere from a few minutes to a few hours. A person who is having a panic attack may experience such physical symptoms as dizziness, trembling, sweating, difficulty breathing, or increased heart rate. He may feel like he is having a heart attack. If panic attacks occur on a regular basis, a person may be diagnosed with panic disorder.

*panic disorder:* A type of anxiety disorder. See Appendix C for details.

*parent–child interaction therapy (PCIT):* A type of therapy that focuses on reducing conflict between the parent and the child, reducing the child's disruptive behaviors, and strengthening the parent–child relationship. Parents are taught new techniques for interacting with their children and then have an opportunity to practice these skills with their children while receiving live coaching, via a headset, from a therapist who is observing the parent–child interactions through a one-way mirror. A related therapy technique, parent–child interaction therapy emotion development (PCITED), which focuses on emotional regulation skills, has been used to treat depression in preschoolers, and hyperactivity and conduct problems in older children.

*personality disorder:* "An enduring pattern of inner experience and behavior that deviates markedly from the expectations of the individual's culture, is pervasive and inflexible, has an onset in adolescence or early adulthood, is stable over time, and leads to distress or impairment," as defined by the American Psychiatric Association. At least 15% of U.S. adults have at least one personality disorder.

*phobia:* An intense fear. Specific phobia is a type of anxiety disorder. See Appendix C for details.

*play therapy:* A type of therapy that encourages children to communicate and solve their problems through play.

*positive behavior support (PBS): See* effective behavior support (EBS).

*posttraumatic stress disorder (PTSD):* A psychological disorder caused by a traumatic event involving actual or threatened death or serious injury to oneself or others. A person suffering from PTSD may experience flashbacks (mental reenactments of the event), emotional numbing, dissociative states, difficulty concentrating, and altered moods.

*prognosis:* The likely outcome of a medical condition.

*protective factor:* Anything that decreases the likelihood that someone will develop a disorder or that helps to reduce the severity of that disorder. *See also* risk factor.

*psychiatrist:* A medical doctor who has received specialized training in psychiatric medicine, which is the branch of medicine that focuses on the prevention, diagnosis, and treatment of mental, emotional, and behavioral disorders.

*psychologist:* A mental health professional who has obtained a doctoral degree in psychology (which the American Psychological Association defines as "the study of the mind and behavior").

*psychosis:* A disturbance in mental functioning in which a person loses touch with reality. A person experiencing psychosis may exhibit changes in thinking patterns, changes in mood, delusions, or hallucinations.

*psychotherapy:* The treatment of mental illness by psychological rather than pharmacological means (medication).

*reactive attachment disorder (RAD):* A mental disorder that is characterized by serious difficulties with attachments to others. It is a severe and rare disorder.

*recovery:* *Recovery* can have two meanings: personal recovery or clinical recovery. *Personal recovery* means learning to live a meaningful and hope-filled life despite the limitations of illness. It is separate and distinct from *clinical recovery*, which refers to medical recovery from illness.

*respite care:* Care that is designed to provide family members and other caregivers with short breaks (or respite) from the day-to-day responsibility of caring for a family member with a mental health problem.

*risk factor:* Anything that increases the likelihood (or risk) that someone will develop a disorder or that increases the severity of that disorder. *See also* protective factor.

*safety plan:* A plan designed to keep everyone, including your child, safe at home, at school, and/or in the community.

*schizophrenia spectrum and other psychotic disorders:* A series of disorders that are characterized by abnormalities in one or more of the following areas: delusions, hallucinations, disorganized thinking or speech, abnormal movement, and disruptions to normal emotions and behaviors (including a lack of emotion). They include schizophrenia, other psychotic disorders, and schizotypal personality disorder.

*self-care:* The act of taking care of your own physical, mental, and emotional well-being.

*self-harm:* When people injure themselves without intending to kill themselves. Sometimes the term *self-injury* is used in place of *self-harm*.

*self-stigma:* When people direct stigma inward. A fear of rejection by others (as a result of stigma) leads some people with mental illness to avoid seeking treatment and to fail to pursue education and employment opportunities. *See also* stigma.

*separation anxiety disorder:* A type of anxiety disorder. See Appendix C for details.

*serotonin:* A neurotransmitter (or "brain messenger") involved in mood, impulsivity, anger, and aggressiveness.

*social phobia:* Also known as *social anxiety disorder.* See Appendix C for details.

*social workers:* Mental health professionals who help people to understand the sources of their problems, to develop coping skills, and to tap into services and supports in their communities.

*special needs:* A term used to describe students who have some sort of disability (intellectual, physical, sensory, emotional, or behavioral), or a learning disability, or who have been identified as gifted.

*stigma:* A form of negative stereotyping that is based on fear and misinformation. Three out of four people with a mental illness report that they have experienced stigma.

*stress:* A state of emotional or mental strain resulting from a real or perceived threat. The body's reaction to that threat.

*substance abuse:* Substance abuse is diagnosed based on the impact that substance use is having on a person's life, for example, whether it's causing problems at school or in relationships, or trouble with the law.

*suicidal ideation:* Having thoughts about suicide.

*trauma:* Any experience causing extreme psychological or physical harm and leading to difficulties with everyday functioning. Psychological trauma at any age can permanently alter the functioning of the brain, resulting in ongoing difficulty.

*treatment plan:* A plan detailing the proposed course of treatment. It acts as a road map for the family and the treatment team.

# Appendix B

# Resources

## BOOKS

You will find an expanded list of recommended readings on the official website for this book: *www.anndouglas.net*.

American Psychiatric Association. *Diagnostic and Statistical Manual of Mental Disorders*. Fifth Edition. Washington, DC: American Psychiatric Publishing, 2013.

Andrews, Debra, and William Mahoney, eds. *Children with School Problems: A Physician's Manual*. Second Edition. Toronto: John Wiley & Sons Canada, Ltd., 2012.

Arden, John B. *Rewire Your Brain: Think Your Way to a Better Life*. Toronto: John Wiley & Sons, 2010.

Barkley, Russell A., and Christine M. Benton. *Your Defiant Child: Eight Steps to Better Behavior*. Second Edition. New York: The Guilford Press, 2013.

Brown, Stuart, with Christopher Vaughan. *Play: How It Shapes the Brain, Opens the Imagination, and Invigorates the Soul*. New York: Penguin Books, 2009.

Craig, Susan E. *Reaching and Teaching Children Who Hurt: Strategies for Your Classroom*. East Peoria, IL: Paul H. Brookes Publishing Co., 2008.

Dweck, Carol S. *Mindset: The New Psychology of Success*. New York: Ballantine Books, 2006.

Dweck, Carol S. *Self-Theories: Their Role in Motivation, Personality, and Development*. New York: Psychology Press, 2000.

Garland, Teresa. *Self-Regulation Interventions and Strategies: Keeping the Body, Mind, and Emotions on Task in Children with Autism, ADHD, or Sensory Disorders*. Eau Claire, WI: PESI Publishing and Media, 2014.

Graham, Linda. *Bouncing Back: Rewiring Your Brain for Maximum Resilience and Well-Being*. Novato, CA: New World Library, 2013.

Greenberger, Dennis, and Christine A. Padesky. *Mind Over Mood: Change How You Feel by Changing the Way You Think*. Second Edition. New York: The Guilford Press, 2015.

Greene, Ross W., and J. Stuart Ablon. *Treating Explosive Kids: The Collaborative Problem-Solving Approach*. New York: The Guilford Press, 2006.

Hall, Karyn D., and Melissa H. Cook. *The Power of Validation: Arming Your Child Against Bullying, Peer Pressure, Addiction, Self-Harm, and Out-of-Control Emotions*. Oakland, CA: New Harbinger Publications, 2012.

Harvey, Pat, and Jeanine A. Penzo. *Parenting a Child Who Has Intense Emotions: Dialectical Behavior Therapy Skills to Help Your Child Regulate Emotional Outbursts and Aggressive Behaviors*. Oakland, CA: New Harbinger Publications, 2009.

Honig, Alice Sterling. *Little Kids, Big Worries: Stress-Busting Tips for Early Childhood Classrooms*. East Peoria, Illinois: Paul H. Brookes Publishing Co., 2010.

Huebner, Dawn. *What to Do When You Worry Too Much*. Washington, DC: Magination Press, 2006.

Huebner, Dawn. *What to Do When Your Temper Flares*. Washington, DC: Magination Press, 2008.

Jensen, Peter S., and Kimberly Eaton Hoagwood, eds. *Improving Children's Mental Health Through Parent Empowerment: A Guide to Assisting Families*. New York: Oxford University Press, 2008.

Karp, David A. *The Burden of Sympathy: How Families Cope with Mental Illness*. New York: Oxford University Press, 2004.

Kashdan, Todd B., and Joseph Ciarrochi, eds. *Mindfulness, Acceptance, and Positive Psychology: The Seven Foundations of Well-Being*. Oakland, CA: Context Press, 2013.

Kemper, Kathi J. *Mental Health, Naturally: The Family Guide to Holistic Care for a Healthy Mind and Body*. Elk Grove Village, IL: American Academy of Pediatrics, 2010.

Koerner, Kelly. *Doing Dialectical Behavior Therapy: A Practical Guide*. New York: The Guilford Press, 2012.

Kuypers, Leah M. *The Zones of Regulation: A Curriculum Designed to Foster Self-Regulation and Emotional Control*. San Jose, CA: Social Thinking Publishing, 2011.

Long, Liza. *The Price of Silence: A Mom's Perspective on Mental Illness*. New York: Plume Books, 2015.

McClelland, Megan M., and Shauna L. Tominey. *Stop, Think, Act: Integrating Self-Regulation in the Early Childhood Classroom*. New York: Routledge, 2015.

McGonigal, Kelly. *The Upside of Stress: Why Stress Is Good for You, and How to Get Good at It*. New York: Avery, 2015.

McGonigal, Kelly. *The Willpower Instinct: How Self-Control Works, Why It Matters, and What You Can Do to Get More of It*. New York: Avery, 2012.

Monti, Daniel A., and Bernard D. Beitman. *Integrative Psychiatry*. Toronto: Oxford University Press, 2010.

Neff, Kristin. *Self-Compassion: Stop Beating Yourself Up and Leave Insecurity Behind*. New York: HarperCollins, 2011.

Neufeld, Gordon, and Gabor Maté. *Hold On to Your Kids: Why Parents Need to Matter More Than Peers*. Toronto: Vintage Canada, 2005.

Ogilvie, Bev. *ConnectZone.org: Building Connectedness in Schools*. Vancouver, BC: Inside Out Media, 2014.

Parker, Helen, Janet Phillips, and Cathy Bedard. *Speaking Up! A Parent Guide to Advocating for Students in Public Schools*. Port Coquitlam, BC: BC Confederation of Parent Advisory Councils, 2008.

Prizant, Barry M., with Tom Fields-Meyer. *Uniquely Human: A Different Way of Seeing Autism*. New York: Simon & Schuster, 2015.

Ratey, John J., with Eric Hagerman. *Spark: The Revolutionary New Science of Exercise and the Brain*. New York: Little, Brown & Co., 2008.

Restak, Richard. *Think Smart: A Neuroscientist's Prescription for Improving Your Brain's Performance*. New York: Riverhead Books, 2009.

Shanker, Stuart. *Calm, Alert, and Learning: Classroom Strategies for Self-Regulation*. Toronto: Pearson Education, 2013.

Siegel, Daniel J., and Tina Payne Bryson. *The Whole-Brain Child: 12 Revolutionary Strategies to Nurture Your Child's Developing Mind*. New York: Delacorte Press, 2011.

Silberman, Steve. *NeuroTribes: The Legacy of Autism and the Future of Neurodiversity*. New York: Avery, 2015.

Slade, Mike. *Personal Recovery and Mental Illness: A Guide for Mental Health Professionals*. New York: Cambridge University Press, 2009.

Solomon, Andrew. *Far from the Tree: Parents, Children, and the Search for Identity*. New York: Scribner, 2012.

Solomon, Andrew. *The Noonday Demon: An Atlas of Depression*. New York: Scribner, 2001.

Southam-Gerow, Michael A. *Emotion Regulation in Children and Adolescents: A Practitioner's Guide*. New York: The Guilford Press, 2013.

Stossel, Scott. *My Age of Anxiety: Fear, Hope, Dread, and the Search for Peace of Mind*. New York: Vintage Books, 2015.

Ungar, Michael. *Too Safe for Their Own Good: How Risk and Responsibility Help Teens Thrive*. Toronto: McClelland & Stewart, 2007.

Van Dijk, Sheri. *Calming the Emotional Storm: Using Dialectical Therapy Skills to Manage Your Emotions and Balance Your Life*. Oakland, CA: New Harbinger Publications, 2012.

Van Dijk, Sheri. *DBT Made Simple: A Step-by-Step Guide to Dialectical Behavior Therapy*. Oakland, CA: New Harbinger Publications, 2012.

Vohs, Kathleen D., and Roy F. Baumeister. *Handbook of Self-Regulation: Research, Theory, and Applications*. Second Edition. New York: The Guilford Press, 2011.

Wilens, Timothy E., and Paul G. Hammerness. *Straight Talk about Psychiatric Medications for Kids*. Fourth Edition. The Guilford Press, 2016.

Woolis, Rebecca. *When Someone You Love Has a Mental Illness: A Handbook for Families, Friends, and Caregivers*. New York: Penguin, 2003.

## Online Resources

What follows is a list of key resources of interest to parents who have a child who is struggling. The official website for this book (*www.anndouglas.net*) features links to additional resources.

### *U.S. Resources*

#### Active Minds

*activeminds.org*

The official website for Active Minds, a nonprofit organization that sparks conversations about mental health on college campuses. The site features a family resources area that will be of interest to parents.

#### ADDitude

*www.additudemag.com*

The website associated with the magazine of the same name, which offers "strategies and support" for individuals living with ADHD and learning disabilities. Features an archive of articles plus access to online support.

#### American Academy of Child and Adolescent Psychiatry

*www.aacap.org*

The official website of the American Academy of Child and Adolescent Psychiatry. Features resources of interest to parents and professionals, including fact sheets, topic-specific resource guides, and a child and adolescent psychiatrist finder search tool.

#### American Academy of Pediatrics

*www.aap.org*

The official website of the American Academy of Pediatrics. Features resources of interest to parents and professionals, including links to *HealthyChildren.org* (the Academy's website for parents).

#### American Psychiatric Association

*www.psych.org*

The official website of the American Psychiatric Association. Features resources of interest to parents and professionals, including comprehensive guides to common mental disorders (symptoms, risk factors, and treatment options) and a "find a psychiatrist" search tool.

## American Psychological Association

*www.apa.org*

The official website of the American Psychological Association. Features a comprehensive Psychology Help Center with articles on parenting, school, and emotional wellness, plus a "psychologist locator" search tool.

## Anxiety and Depression Association of America

*www.adaa.org*

The official website of the Anxiety and Depression Association of America, a national nonprofit organization dedicated to the prevention, treatment, and cure of anxiety and mood disorders, OCD, and PTSD. Features articles on living and thriving with a mood disorder plus a "find a therapist" search tool.

## Association for Applied Psychophysiology and Biofeedback

*www.aapb.org*

The official website of the Association for Applied Psychophysiology and Biofeedback—a nonprofit research organization. Features advice on choosing a practitioner and distinguishing between evidence-based and nonevidence forms of treatment.

## Autism Society of America

*www.autism-society.org*

The official website of the Autism Society of America, a national grassroots association that focuses on education and advocacy. Provides practical advice on living with autism, including advice for family members, as well as research updates.

## The Balanced Mind Parent Network

*www.thebalancedmind.org*

The Balanced Mind Parent Network (BMPN), a program of the Depression and Bipolar Support Alliance (DBSA), offers guidance and support to families raising children with mood disorders, including information about accessing both in-person and online support groups.

## Bazelon Center for Mental Health Law

*www.bazelon.org*

A national nonprofit that advocates for the rights of children and adults with mental disabilities. A comprehensive website featuring in-depth legal resources and policy documents.

**Bipolar Disorder Magazine**

*www.bphope.com*

The website associated with the magazine of the same name. Features a selection of articles and blog posts from people living with bipolar disorder.

**Brain & Behavior Research Foundation**

*http://bbrfoundation.org*

The official website of the Brain & Behavior Research Foundation, which funds research into the causes and treatment of a variety of mental disorders. The website features research updates as well as stories of people who are living with mental illness.

**Bring Change 2 Mind**

*www.bringchange2mind.org*

A nonprofit organization cofounded by actress Glenn Close to combat the stigma associated with mental illness. Features first-person accounts of mental illness plus opportunities for online advocacy.

**Center for Early Childhood Mental Health Consultation**

*http://ecmhc.org*

Part of the Georgetown University Center for Child and Human Development, the Center for Early Childhood Mental Consultation website features resources of interest to parents and professionals. The materials for families include stress management resources and advice on promoting the healthy social and emotional development of young children.

**Center for Effective Collaboration and Practice**

*http://cecp.air.org*

The official website of the Center for Effective Collaboration and Practice, a national umbrella organization connecting organizations that are working to help children living with or at risk of developing serious emotional disorders.

**Center on Early Adolescence**

*www.earlyadolescence.org*

The Center on Early Adolescence is a national research organization funded by the National Institute on Drug Abuse. It focuses on the "development, treatment, and prevention of problems of early adolescence" by encouraging the development of nurturing environments for young people. The website features practical, evidence-based articles on parenting practices that encourage children to thrive.

## Center on the Social and Emotional Foundations for Early Learning

*csefel.vanderbilt.edu*

The Center on the Social and Emotional Foundations for Early Learning is a national resource center aimed at promoting the social emotional development and school readiness of young children. The website features a series of "family tools" tip sheets focusing on such topics as emotional literacy and relationship skills.

## Children and Adults with Attention-Deficit/Hyperactivity Disorder

*www.chadd.org*

Children and Adults with Attention-Deficit/Hyperactivity Disorder (CHADD) is a national membership organization founded in response to the "frustration and sense of isolation" experienced by parents of children with ADHD. Features practical advice and advocacy information as well as a directory of ADHD-related support groups and professional services.

## Child Mind Institute

*www.childmind.org*

A comprehensive website associated with the New York City–based clinic of the same name. Features a wealth of resources related to mental health and learning disorders, including a practical guide to accessing and navigating treatment ("Parents Guide to Getting Good Care").

## Council for Exceptional Children

*www.cec.sped.org*

The official website of the Council for Exceptional Children, which bills itself as "the largest international professional organization dedicated to improving the educational success of individuals with disabilities and/or gifts and talents." A good starting point for anyone researching special education rights and advocacy issues.

## Depression and Bipolar Support Alliance

*www.dbsalliance.org*

A national peer support network focused on improving the lives of people living with depression or bipolar disorder. Offers practical advice plus peer support (both in person and online).

## International OCD Foundation

*www.ocfoundation.org*

A nonprofit organization that focuses on improving the lives of people living with obsessive–compulsive disorder. Features advice for parents and for kids as well as a comprehensive directory of services and supports.

## Juvenile Bipolar Research Foundation

*www.jbrf.org*

The Juvenile Bipolar Research Foundation is a nonprofit that funds research into the causes and treatment of bipolar disorder in children. The website features research updates and practical advice on advocating for your child at school.

## LD Online: Learning Disabilities and ADHD

*www.ldonline.org*

One of the oldest and most established websites focusing on learning disabilities and ADHD. Features expert advice and personal stories.

## Learning Disabilities Association of America

*www.ldanatl.org*

The official website of the Learning Disabilities Association of America, a nonprofit education and advocacy organization. Comprehensive resources on education law plus practical guides to becoming a powerful advocate for your child.

## National Alliance on Mental Illness

*www.nami.org*

The official website of the National Alliance on Mental Illness—a massive grass-roots education and advocacy organization working on behalf of individuals and families living with mental illness. Offers comprehensive and practical resources as well as access to peer-led support groups and a national support helpline.

## National Center for Learning Disabilities

*www.ncld.org*

A national advocacy organization that seeks to improve the lives of the one in five children and adults living with a learning disability or attention issue. Offers resources of interest to parents, educators, professionals, and children/teens.

## National Center for Mental Health and Juvenile Justice

*www.ncmhjj.com*

An organization that advocates on behalf of "justice-involved" youth, with an emphasis on meeting the needs of young people with mental health issues who are at risk of or end up being incarcerated.

## National Council on Disability

*www.ncd.gov*

The official website of the National Council on Disability, a federal agency that is responsible for advising the federal government about "policies, programs, practices, and procedures that affect people with disabilities." A helpful resource for questions related to disability law.

### National Federation of Families for Children's Mental Health

*www.ffcmh.org*

A national organization focusing on the needs of children and youth with emotional, behavioral, or mental health issues as well as the needs of their families. Features parenting advice and links to resources and supports at the state and local level.

### National Institute of Mental Health

*www.nimh.nih.gov*

The official website of the National Institute of Mental Health, the leading federal agency for research on mental disorders. Includes a wealth of resources related to child and adolescent mental health and practical advice on accessing treatment.

### Selective Mutism Group: Childhood Anxiety Network

*www.selectivemutism.org*

A nonprofit organization that focuses on providing information and support to families with a child who is struggling with the anxiety disorder known as selective mutism (SM). Features a directory of support groups, advice on accessing treatment, and an online library featuring articles on a variety of mental health, parenting, and education-related topics.

### Understood.org

*www.understood.org*

A comprehensive and parent-friendly resource created by a consortium of 15 nonprofit organizations, including the Child Mind Institute, the Learning Disabilities Association of America, and the National Center for Learning Disabilities. You'll find articles, tip sheets, and advocacy resources galore. A truly outstanding resource.

## *Selected International Resources*

### Autism Research Centre

*www.autismresearchcentre.com*

A U.K.-based research center that focuses on the biomedical causes of autism. The site features research updates and links to autism research organizations worldwide.

### CanChild Centre for Childhood Disability Research

*www.canchild.ca*

A Canadian research center that focuses on studying children and youth with developmental disabilities as well as their families. Features disability-specific resource guides as well as advice for practitioners on providing family-centered care.

## Centre for Clinical Interventions

*www.cci.health.wa.gov.au*

An Australian mental health agency that delivers evidence-based programs (and that trains health care providers in the delivery of evidence-based programs) for anxiety disorders, mood disorders, and eating disorders. In the consumer resources section of the website, you'll find downloadable guides to managing moods, overcoming perfectionism, and other related topics.

## Children of Parents with a Mental Illness

*www.copmi.net.au*

A family support initiative funded by the Australian government. The website features resources for parents (on parenting while living with a mental illness), children, and youth (about supporting a parent who is living with a mental illness), as well as related resources for extended family members, friends, and professionals.

## Embrace the Future Resiliency Resource Centre

*www.embracethefuture.org.au*

A youth mental health project initiated by the Mental Health Foundation of Australia. The project seeks to educate young people up to the age of 24 in "strategies and skills which promote and sustain resiliency and positive mental health." The website features materials for children, youth, and parents/educators.

## Headspace

*www.headspace.org.au*

Headspace is Australia's national youth mental health foundation. It focuses on early intervention services for young people between the ages of 12 and 25. The organization's website features a parent information area with information about adolescent development, parenting strategies, and the warning signs of mental illness.

## Institute of Families for Child and Youth Mental Health

*www.familysmart.ca*

A Canadian nonprofit organization that involves children, youth, and families in designing mental health care systems and establishing standards of mental health care. The website features resources related to family-friendly mental health care services and family engagement.

## Mental Health Foundation

*www.mentalhealth.org.uk*

A U.K.-based charity that emphasizes research and that seeks to influence mental health policy making. The website features a wealth of resources on a wide variety of mental health issues, including child and youth mental health, mindfulness, and self-care.

## Mind

*www.mind.org.uk*

A U.K.-based charity focused on education and the eradication of stigma. The organization's website features a library of downloadable resources on a range of mental health topics, including self-care for family members.

## National Autistic Society

*autism.org.uk*

A U.K.-based charity for people with autism spectrum disorders. Features articles on living with or supporting a family member with autism, including a comprehensive collection of resources for and about siblings.

## YoungMinds

*www.youngminds.org.uk*

A U.K.-based charity that is focused on improving the emotional well-being and mental health of children and young people. The website contains numerous resources of interest to parents, including information about common mental health and behavior concerns in children and youth and advice on parenting strategies.

# Appendix C

# Directory of Disorders

What follows is basic information about some of the more commonly diagnosed mental, neurodevelopmental, and behavioral disorders in children and adolescents. For additional information about these and other disorders, please consult the official website for this book, *www.anndouglas.net*, as well as the other two appendices.

### Attention-Deficit/Hyperactivity Disorder (ADHD)

*Incidence:* 5% of children and 2.5% of adults.

*Typical age of onset:* Childhood. A World Health Organization study narrowed down the typical age of onset to 7 to 9 years of age. ADHD is more likely to occur in males than in females. (The ratio of male to female children is 2:1.)

*Symptoms:* Inattention (wandering off task, lacking persistence, having difficulty sustaining focus, being disorganized); hyperactivity (excessive movement or fidgeting at inappropriate times); impulsivity (hasty actions that occur in the moment without forethought and that have high potential for harm to the individual); an inability to delay gratification; social intrusiveness. Symptoms must be present in more than one setting (for example, at home and at school) in order for a diagnosis to be made. There are three separate subtypes of ADHD: the primarily hyperactive–impulsive subtype (which is quite rare), the primarily inattentive subtype (formerly known as *attention deficit disorder*), and the combined subtype (the most common type of ADHD, which is made up of individuals who exhibit symptoms of hyperactivity, impulsivity, and inattention).

*Other conditions that may be found in someone with this diagnosis:* Mild delays in language, motor, or social development; difficulties with executive function or memory; specific learning disorder; anxiety disorders; major depressive disorder; obsessive–compulsive disorder; tic disorders; and autism spectrum

259

disorder. Conduct disorder occurs in about one-quarter of children and adolescents with the combined subtype of ADHD. The risk of suicide increases by early adulthood if a diagnosis of ADHD is also accompanied by a mood, conduct, or substance use disorder.

### Autism Spectrum Disorder (ASD)

*Incidence*: 1% of the population.

*Typical age of onset*: Symptoms are typically recognized in early childhood.

*Symptoms*: Persistent impairment in reciprocal social communication and social interaction, and restricted, repetitive patterns of behavior, interest, or activities. These symptoms are present from early childhood and limit or impair everyday functioning.

*Other conditions that may be found in someone with this diagnosis*: Intellectual impairment, language disorders, attention-deficit/hyperactivity disorder, developmental coordination disorder, anxiety disorders, depressive disorders. Approximately 70% of people with ASD have a psychiatric disorder, and about 40% of people with ASD have two or more psychiatric disorders.

### Bipolar and Related Disorders

*Incidence*: 2.7% in adolescents; no statistics are available for younger children.

*Typical age of onset*: Childhood, adolescence, adulthood.

*Symptoms*: Mood disturbances that are extreme enough to disrupt a person's life. For a diagnosis of bipolar I to be made, a person must have experienced at least one manic episode. For a diagnosis of bipolar II to be made, a person must have experienced a current or past hypomanic episode and a current or past depressive episode.

*Other conditions that may be found in someone with this diagnosis*: Anxiety disorders, substance use disorders, eating disorders (binge-eating disorder is the most common).

## Anxiety Disorders (in Order of Typical Age of Onset)

### Separation Anxiety

*Incidence:* 4% of children and 1.6% of adolescents.

*Typical age of onset:* Childhood.

*Symptoms:* Fearfulness or anxiety about separation from parents that is much greater than what is typically experienced by other children the same age (excessive "clinginess"). The child may worry about harm coming to his parents. This may lead to nightmares and physical symptoms of distress.

*Other conditions that may be found in someone with this diagnosis:* Generalized anxiety disorder and specific phobia.

## Selective Mutism

*Incidence:* Relatively rare.

*Typical age of onset:* Prior to age 5.

*Symptoms:* A consistent failure to speak in social situations or in situations in which there is an expectation that the child will speak (for example, when the child has been asked to give a speech at school). The failure to speak is interfering with the child's ability to perform at school or to engage in social interactions.

*Other conditions that may be found in someone with this diagnosis:* Other anxiety disorders, communication delays or disorders.

## Specific Phobia

*Incidence:* 5% of children and 16% of 13- to 17-year-olds; females are twice as likely to experience specific phobias as males.

*Typical age of onset:* Childhood and adolescence.

*Symptoms:* A fear or anxiety about a particular object or situation that is out of proportion to the actual risk involved.

*Other conditions that may be found in someone with this diagnosis:* Other anxiety disorders, mood disorders, disruptive behavior disorders.

## Social Anxiety Disorders

*Incidence:* 7% of children and adults.

*Typical age of onset:* Ages 8 to 15.

*Symptoms:* A fear or anxiety about social situations. The child may be particularly anxious about meeting unfamiliar people or having to perform in front of others, and fear risking potential humiliation or rejection.

*Other conditions that may be found in someone with this diagnosis:* Other anxiety disorders, major depressive disorder, substance use disorders, body dysmorphic disorder, high-functioning autism.

## Panic Disorder

*Incidence:* 2 to 3% of adolescents and adults.

*Typical age of onset:* Ages 20 to 24 years.

*Symptoms:* A condition that can occur after a child has experienced a panic attack. She becomes fearful of experiencing another panic attack and goes to great lengths to avoid any situation that could leave her vulnerable (for example, being on her own in public).

*Other conditions that may be found in someone with this diagnosis*: Other anxiety disorders, major depressive disorder, bipolar disorder.

## Generalized Anxiety Disorder (GAD)

*Incidence*: 0.9% of adolescents.

*Typical age of onset*: Varies widely.

*Symptoms*: Persistent and excessive anxiety and worry that carry over into multiple areas of a person's life. GAD is characterized by restlessness, edginess, difficulty concentrating, fatigue, muscle tension, and sleep disturbances.

*Other conditions that may be found in someone with this diagnosis*: Other anxiety disorders and other depressive disorders.

## Obsessive–Compulsive Disorder (OCD)

*Incidence*: 1.2%; during childhood, males are more likely to be affected.

*Typical age of onset*: 25% of cases begin before age 14. Males have an earlier age of onset than females, with 25% of cases beginning before age 10.

*Symptoms*: The presence of obsessions (recurrent and persistent thoughts, urges, or images that are intrusive and unwanted) and compulsions (repetitive behaviors or mental acts that a person feels driven to perform in response to an obsession).

*Other conditions that may be found in someone with this diagnosis*: Other anxiety disorders, depressive or bipolar disorders, tic disorders.

## Depressive Disorders

### Major Depressive Disorder (MDD)

*Incidence*: 7%; the incidence of MDD in females as compared to males is one and a half to three times higher, starting in early adolescence.

*Typical age of onset*: May appear at any age, but the likelihood of onset peaks at puberty.

*Symptoms*: Depressed mood (irritability or sadness), fatigue, sleep disturbance, appetite changes, increased agitation or a loss of energy, a loss of interest in nearly all activities, feelings of worthlessness or guilt, difficulty concentrating, thoughts of death.

*Other conditions that may be found in someone with this diagnosis*: Substance use disorder, panic disorder, obsessive–compulsive disorder, anorexia nervosa, bulimia nervosa, and borderline personality disorder.

## Disruptive Mood Dysregulation Disorder

*Incidence*: 2 to 5% of children and adolescents.

*Typical age of onset*: Prior to age 10.

*Symptoms*: Chronic, severe, persistent irritability, and marked disruption to relationships and school performance. Dangerous behavior, suicide ideation, suicide attempts, and severe aggression are common.

*Other conditions that may be found in someone with this diagnosis*: Disruptive behavior disorders (especially oppositional defiant disorder), mood disorder, anxiety disorders, autism spectrum disorder.

# Disruptive, Impulse Control, and Conduct Disorders

## Oppositional Defiant Disorder (ODD)

*Incidence*: 3.3%; it's four times as common in males as in females prior to adolescence.

*Typical age of onset*: Preschool age.

*Symptoms*: A frequent and persistent pattern of angry or irritable mood, argumentative and defiant behavior, or vindictiveness.

*Other conditions that may be found in someone with this diagnosis*: Attention-deficit/ hyperactivity disorder, anxiety disorders, major depressive disorder, substance use disorder, and conduct disorder.

## Conduct Disorder

*Incidence*: 4%.

*Typical age of onset*: Childhood and adolescence. Prevalence rates rise from childhood to adolescence.

*Symptoms*: A repetitive and persistent pattern of behavior in which the basic rights of others are violated. If conduct disorder emerges during childhood as opposed to adolescence, physical aggression toward others and disturbed peer relationships are typical. If conduct disorder emerges during adolescence, it tends to be less severe in nature.

*Other conditions that may be found in someone with this diagnosis*: Attention-deficit/ hyperactivity disorder, oppositional defiant disorder, specific learning disorder, anxiety disorders, depressive or bipolar disorders.

# Index

Index

# About the Author

Ann Douglas is an award-winning parenting writer and the mother of four children who have struggled with a variety of psychological problems—and are currently thriving.

She speaks widely at health, parenting, and education conferences and hosts online conversations about parenting and mental health for a range of organizations.

With acclaimed books including *The Mother of All Parenting Books* and *The Mother of All Baby Books*, Ann has helped hundreds of thousands of parents navigate the challenges and complexities of raising kids today. She lives with her husband and their youngest child in Peterborough, Ontario.